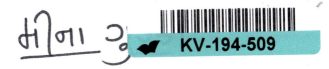

RADIOGRAPHIC TECHNIQUES RELATED TO PATHOLOGY

Radiographic Techniques related to Pathology

BY

MARGARET A. CLIFFORD DCR
Radiographer,
Lord Mayor Treloers Hospital,
Alton, Hants

AND

ANN E. DRUMMOND BA, FCR
District Superintendent Radiographer,
Frimley Park Hospital,
Frimley, Surrey

WITH A FOREWORD BY

T. H. HILLS MB, DMRE
Director, X-ray Department, Guy's Hospital, London

Third Edition

WRIGHT · P S G

BRISTOL LONDON BOSTON
1983

Published by
John Wright & Sons Ltd, 823—825 Bath Road, Bristol
BS4 5NU, England.
John Wright PSG Inc., 545 Great Road, Littleton,
Massachusetts 01460, U.S.A.

First edition, 1968
Second edition, 1977
Reprinted, 1981
Third edition, 1983

British Library Cataloguing in Publication Data
Clifford, Margaret
    Radiographic techniques related to pathology.
    3rd ed.
    1. Diagnosis, Radioscopic
    I. Title   II. Drummond, Ann E.
    616.07'57   RC78

ISBN 0 7236 0679 X

Library of Congress Catalog Card Number: 83—42671

Printed in Great Britain by
John Wright & Sons Printing Ltd at The Stonebridge Press,
Bristol

Preface to the Third Edition

In this new edition we have not changed our aim of providing a pocket guide for radiographers where full-time radiological advice is not available. We have, however, made additions and some amendments where new techniques have become available.

Only basic techniques are included and the views suggested are guidelines and can be adjusted to suit radiological preferences. In many cases, more extensive or specialized examinations, including fluoroscopy, the use of opaque media, radio-nuclide imaging or ultrasound, may be necessary. With the exception of the latter, these have not been included as they may only be requested and supervised by a qualified medical practitioner.

We have compiled a short Appendix to cover some specialized techniques, a list of projections covering skeletal survey and bone age, etc. Also included are some generally used abbreviations.

We wish to express our thanks to Dr T. H. Hills, Director of the X-ray Department at Guy's Hospital; Dr D. Pocock, Lecturer in Forensic Medicine at St George's Hospital; Dr A. W. Simmins, Consultant Radiologist at Heatherwood Hospital, Ascot; and Dr R. O. Murray, Consultant Orthopaedic Radiologist at Heatherwood Hospital, for all their assistance in the revision of this handbook, and to all our other friends and colleagues for their support and encouragement, and also those who have aided us with the revised 3rd edition.

Foreword

By T. H. HILLS MB, DMRE

Director, X-ray Department, Guy's Hospital, London

TAKING a good-quality radiograph requires a combination of sound training, experience, and an intelligent appreciation of the problems involved. The routine work of most radiographers is largely unsupervised, and without any knowledge of the disease process it may be difficult to know if the films taken are the best demonstration of an abnormality if present.

Sometimes additional views besides the standard projections are of great value, and if the radiographer, after inspection of a film, can with confidence realize what more is required for diagnostic purposes, the patient may well be saved another visit to the hospital.

The use of this comprehensive work will certainly enable the intelligent radiographer to take a greater and more informed interest in his/her patients with the production of valuable radiographs.

Throughout this text the abbreviations AP and PA stand for antero-posterior and postero-anterior, respectively.

Some commonly used Abbreviations on Request Forms

ALL	Acute lymphatic leukaemia
AS	Ankylosing spondylitis or aortic stenosis
ASD	Atrial septal defect
BNO	Bladder neck obstruction
CCF	Chronic cardiac failure
CDH	Congenital dislocated hip
CNS	Central nervous system
COLD	Chronic obstructive lung/airway disease
CSF	Cerebrospinal fluid
CVA	Cerebrovascular accident
DLE	Disseminated lupus erythematosus
EN	Erythema nodosum
ESN	Educationally sub-normal
ESR	Erythrocyte sedimentation rate
FTND	Full term normal delivery
IDK	Internal derangement of the knee joint
IHD	Ischaemic heart disease
IUD	Intra uterine device
LE	Lupus erythematosus
LMP	Last menstrual period
MA	Mental age
MBC	Maximum breathing capacity
MD	Mentally deficient
MS	Multiple sclerosis or mitral stenosis
OA	Osteoarthritis
PD	Peritoneal dialysis
PE	Pulmonary embolism
PID	Prolapsed inter-vertebral disc
RA	Rheumatoid arthritis
ROM	Range of movement
SBE	Sub bacterial endocarditis
SED	Skin erythema dose
SFD	Signs of fetal death/distress
SM	Systolic murmur
SOL	Space occupying lesion
TB	Tuberculosis
THR	Total hip replacement
TIA	Transient ischaemic attack
TKR	Total knee replacement
VD	Venereal disease
VDH	Valvular disease of the heart

Radiographic Techniques related to Pathology

ACHALASIA OF THE CARDIA (Cardiospasm)
The oesophagus is dilated due to impairment of muscle contraction and inability of the cardiac sphincter to open properly.
TECHNIQUE
PA chest.
Penetrated PA chest—increase 10 kV.
Penetrated lateral.

ACHONDROPLASIA
Congenital impairment of the endochondral ossification leading to extreme shortness and flaring of the metaphyses of the long bones. Failure of the neural arch to develop, resulting in narrowing of the neural canal. Similarly, the pelvic inlet is small as a result of diminished growth.
TECHNIQUE
AP long bones, including clavicles.
AP and lateral lumbar spine.
AP pelvis.
Lateral skull—to show shortness of the base.

ACOUSTIC NEUROMA
A tumour of the 8th cranial nerve. There may be enlargement of the internal auditory meatus.
TECHNIQUE
AP skull with $25°$, $30°$, and $35°$ caudal tilts.
Stenver's projection—*see* APPENDIX.
Lateral skull.
Submento-vertical projection.

ACROCEPHALOSYNDACTYLIA
See APERT'S SYNDROME.

ACROMEGALY

Overactivity of the eosinophil cells of the anterior lobe of the pituitary gland, usually due to a tumour. It arises in adult life after completion of bone growth, causing some bone enlargement and a coarsening of features.

TECHNIQUE

Lateral skull—to show enlarged frontals and mandible with separation of teeth.

PA hands—to include terminal phalangeal tufts which become much expanded.

Lateral heels soft tissue—to show thickened heel pad.

ACTINOMYCOSIS

A chronic suppurative infection of the tissues by a fungus-like organism, primarily affecting the face, jaws, intestine, lungs, and sometimes bones.

TECHNIQUE

Lateral oblique mandible.

PA chest.

AP affected area.

Lateral affected area.

ADAMANTINOMA (Ameloblastoma)

A rare, slow growing tumour of the mandible. It occurs mainly in males in middle life and involves loosening of the teeth, pain and ulcerations in the mouth. It can also occur in the long bones, the most likely being the tibia.

TECHNIQUE

Lateral obliques of both mandibles—to demonstrate molar region.

ADDISON'S DISEASE

Bilateral hypofunction of the suprarenal cortex, often due to tuberculous infection. Symptoms appear after some 80 per cent of destruction, causing extreme weakness, low blood-pressure, and pigmentation of the skin.

TECHNIQUE

AP upper abdomen—to include diaphragms.

See also SUPRARENAL CALCIFICATION.

ADENOIDS, enlargement of

A swelling of the lymphoid tissue in the nasopharynx, due to recurrent infection.

TECHNIQUE
Lateral nasopharynx using Valsalva's manœuvre,
see APPENDIX.
For children the Valsalva manœuvre is difficult.
Older children are allowed to breathe slowly
through nose with mouth shut.
Young children to have parents place finger under
chin and pinch nose gently.

ALBRIGHT'S NEPHROCALCINOSIS
A dysfunction of the renal tubules causing acids to
accumulate in the blood; the urine contains exces-
sive amounts of calcium, small deposits of which
may be found in the medulla of the kidney.
TECHNIQUE
AP abdomen.
Lateral abdomen—for differential diagnosis.

ALBRIGHT'S SYNDROME
A combination of precocious sexual and skeletal
maturation, plus pigmentation of the skin and
fibrous dysplasia.
TECHNIQUE
Lateral skull—to demonstrate pituitary fossa.
PA hand and wrist—to determine bone age.
AP affected area—to show deformity.
Lateral affected area—to show deformity.

ANAEMIA
A lack of haemoglobin or red cells, or a combination
of both, in the blood. There are many types of
anaemia, but in all cases there is a decrease in the
oxygen content of the blood causing tiredness,
pallor, and shortness of breath.
TECHNIQUE
PA chest.
AP abdomen.

ANENCEPHALY
Failure of the fetal brain to develop, with associated
lack of formation of the bones of the vault of the
skull.
TECHNIQUE
Ultrasound is used for the primary diagnosis
followed by
PA abdomen }
Lateral abdomen } for confirmation.

ANEURYSMAL BONE CYST

A process of disturbance of the vasculature, commencing within cancellous or medullary tissue, eroding the cortex from within, causing an expanding lesion. The outline is similar to that of a saccular aneurysm of the aorta—hence its name. It can occur in any bone, though some 25 per cent of occurrences are in the vertebrae.

TECHNIQUE

AP and lateral of area concerned.

ANGINA PECTORIS

A condition of the heart where the coronary arteries are narrowed and consequently supply insufficient oxygenated blood to the heart muscle. This condition is usually caused by atheromatous deposits in the vessels and causes pain in the chest and left arm during effort.

TECHNIQUE

PA chest at 2 m—for heart size.

ANKYLOSING SPONDYLITIS (Spondylitis Ankylopoetica)

A chronic inflammatory condition involving the spinal ligaments, the most common site of onset being the sacro-iliac joints and the lower lumbar spine.

TECHNIQUE

AP sacro-iliac joints.
Oblique sacro-iliac joints.
AP whole spine.
Lateral whole spine.

AORTIC ANEURYSM

A localized dilatation of the aorta.

1. **Thoracic Aorta**

Some of these are syphilitic in origin.

TECHNIQUE

PA chest.
Lateral chest.
Lateral dorsal spine—to show erosion of anterior border of vertebral bodies.
Right and left obliques with fine focus grid or Potter-Bucky.

2. **Abdominal Aorta**

The majority of these are arteriosclerotic in origin.

TECHNIQUE
>   Ultrasound.
>   AP abdomen——to show extent of aneurysm and whether it is leaking into the psoas muscle.
>   Lateral abdomen—to demonstrate soft tissues.

AORTIC STENOSIS
Narrowing of the aortic valves, often due to atheromatous deposition of the valve cusps.
>   TECHNIQUE
>   PA chest at 2 m—for heart size, and size and shape of aorta, calcified aortic valve may be present.

APERT'S SYNDROME (Acrocephalosyndactylia)
A premature fusion of the skull suture producing a peaked appearance and associated with webbing of the hands and feet.
>   TECHNIQUE
>   AP/PA skull
>   AP feet and PA hands
>   } and high kV low mAs technique to demonstrate soft tissue and bone formation.

ARACHNODACTYLY (Spider Fingers or Marfan's Syndrome)
A condition in which the fingers and toes are unusually long and slender and there is also unusual flexibility of the joints. It is often associated with spina bifida occulta and may be due to increased endochondral ossification——the opposite of achondroplasia.
>   TECHNIQUE
>   PA chest—congenital heart disease is common.
>   PA hands.
>   AP feet.
>   AP thoracic and lumbar spine——to show increased neural canal.
>   Lateral thoracic and lumbar spine.

ARTIFICIAL PNEUMOTHORAX
See PNEUMOTHORAX.

ASSMANN'S FOCUS
Tuberculous manifestation forming a round focus in the apical and subclavicular regions.
>   TECHNIQUE
>   PA chest.
>   Apical view.
>   Tomography.

ATELECTASIS

Areas of collapse of the lung, being either lobar, segmental, or lobular.

TECHNIQUE

PA chest.

Lateral chest.

Posterior oblique chest.

Tomography—if required.

ATHEROSCLEROSIS OF THE AORTA

A degenerative condition of the aorta caused by a patchy deposit of lipoid causing thickening of the walls and narrowing of the lumen.

Frequently linear-shaped areas of calcification appear.

TECHNIQUE

PA chest.

Left anterior oblique chest.

Left lateral chest.

ATRIAL SEPTAL DEFECT (Patent Interauricular Defect)

A congenital heart fault, whereby there is a patent defect of the septum between the two auricles causing breathlessness, but no cyanosis.

TECHNIQUE

PA chest.

AP chest supine in the new born.

Left lateral.

AURICULAR FIBRILLATION

An abnormality of heart rhythm that frequently occurs in right or left ventricular failure. This may cause enlargement of the heart, pulmonary oedema, and pleural effusion.

TECHNIQUE

PA chest at 2 m—for heart size.

Lateral chest.

AZYGOS LOBE

An accessory lobe formed in the apex of the right lung when the azygos vein fails to shift medially during fetal life. It cuts into the right upper lobe leaving a deep pulmonary fissure and is of little clinical significance.

TECHNIQUE
PA chest.
Right anterior oblique chest with only slight rotation.

BAKER'S CYST
See POPLITEAL BURSITIS.

BAMBOO SPINE
See ANKYLOSING SPONDYLITIS.

BANKART'S LESION
A compression defect on the articular surface of the humeral head due to impingement on the edge of the glenoid fossa during dislocation.
TECHNIQUE
See DISLOCATION OF THE SHOULDER—RECURRENT.

BASOPHIL ADENOMA
See CUSHING'S SYNDROME.

BATTERED BABY SYNDROME
See NON-ACCIDENTAL INJURY.

BESNIER-BOECK DISEASE
See SARCOIDOSIS.

BICIPITAL TENDINITIS
See CALCAREOUS TENDINITIS.

BILHARZIASIS
See SCHISTOSOMIASIS.

BLOCK VERTEBRA
Incomplete segmentation of the vertebrae, with partial or complete absence of the intervening discs. This is a congenital anomaly occurring in any part of the spine. The antero-posterior diameter of the affected bodies is diminished, unlike the end-result of fusion from an old infective lesion, with the exception of Still's disease.
TECHNIQUE
AP spine.
Lateral spine.

BLOUNT'S DISEASE (Osteochondritis Deformans Tibiae)

Non-rachitic bowing of the tibiae in children. There is breaking and enlargement of the medial tibial condyle, which usually corrects spontaneously.

TECHNIQUE

AP both knees—to include distal half of femora and proximal half of tibiae.

BORNHOLM'S DISEASE

See EPIDEMIC PLEURODYNIA.

BRACHYDACTYLIA

A congenital deformity of the hands and/or the feet causing abnormal shortness of one or more of the metacarpals and/or the metatarsals.

TECHNIQUE

PA both hands.

AP both feet.

BRACHYPHALANGIA

A congenital deformity resulting in abnormal shortness in one or more of the phalanges, the middle phalanx being more commonly affected.

TECHNIQUE

PA both hands.

AP both feet.

BRODIE'S ABSCESS

A chronic osteomyelitic focus in bone often near the end of a long bone, the abscess formation causing an increase in the density of the cortex. It presents a translucent area surrounded by a zone of density due to reactive sclerosis around the focus of chronic infection.

TECHNIQUE

AP infected area—to include a joint, increase 5–10 kV.

Lateral infected area—to include a joint, increase 5–10 kV.

BRONCHIAL ASTHMA

A generalized obstruction of bronchi by thick secretions; often there is an allergic cause.

TECHNIQUE

PA chest—a reduction in exposure is necessary in chronic cases.

BRONCHIAL CARCINOMA
A malignant tumour mainly arising out of the larger bronchi near the root of the lung.

TECHNIQUE
PA chest.
Lateral chest.
Penetrated PA chest—for visualization of the bronchi.

BRONCHIECTASIS
A dilatation of the bronchi, either local or generalized, the lower lobes being more usually affected. Infection is always present.

TECHNIQUE
PA chest.
Lateral chest ⎫
Oblique chest ⎬ According to the site of disease.
Lordotic view ⎭

BRONCHITIS
An inflammatory condition of the bronchi which can be acute or chronic.

TECHNIQUE
PA chest.

BROWN TUMOUR
A giant-cell-type tumour associated with hyperparathyroidism causing focal areas of bone destruction.

TECHNIQUE
See HYPERPARATHYROIDISM.

BRUCELLOSIS (Malta Fever, Undulant Fever)
A remittent febrile disease contracted from animals. It may cause destruction of the bone and intervening discs of the spine. There may also be moderate enlargement of the spleen, endocarditis followed by congestive heart failure.

TECHNIQUE
AP affected area ⎫ The most common site
Lateral affected area ⎬ being the lower dorsal and
upper lumbar spine.
PA chest—for heart size.
AP abdomen—for enlargement of spleen.

BUMPER FRACTURE
Depressed fracture of the tibial articular surface, due to the impact from the bumper of a car.

TECHNIQUE
AP knee-joint.
Lateral knee-joint—with horizontal beam to demonstrate possible fluid levels.

CACOSMIA (Parosmia)

A perversion of the sense of smell, which may be associated with organic brain disease or psychoneurotic conditions.
TECHNIQUE
Occipito-mental sinuses view.
Lateral skull—to include sinuses.

CAFFEY'S DISEASE (Infantile Cortical Hyperostosis)

A self-limiting disease of infantile cortical hyperostosis. Radiologically it appears as a marked proliferation of bone by the periosteum. The flat bones, mandibles, clavicles, and shaft of long bones are the most frequent sites. The disease usually appears in the first 6 months of life, the bone changes usually appearing when the acute phase of the disease is subsiding.
TECHNIQUE
Lateral skull to include mandibles.
AP mandible.
AP both shoulders—one film to include clavicles and scapulae.
AP pelvis and femora.

CAISSON DISEASE (Decompression Sickness)

A disease caused by over-rapid decompression from high atmospheric pressures. Bubbles of nitrogen are liberated into the blood stream causing a condition known as 'the bends'. The bubbles of nitrogen may block capillaries and cause avascular necrosis of the bone. Radiological changes in the bone may occur several years after an acute episode and occur most frequently in the distal femoral or proximal tibial diaphyses and in the head and neck of the humeri or femora. Lesions have a marked tendency to symmetry.
TECHNIQUE
AP both shoulders.
AP both hips.
AP both knees.

CALCANEAL SPUR
A condition where a bony spur develops on the plantar surface of the calcaneus; it may be uni- or bilateral.
TECHNIQUE
Lateral both heels.

CALCANEO-NAVICULAR BAR
A bridge or bar between the calcaneus and navicular.
TECHNIQUE
Dorsiplantar oblique of the tarsus.
Axial view of the calcaneus—increase 10 kV.

CALCANEUS ACCESSORUS
Said to occur as an epiphysis for the peroneal tubercle of the calcaneus.
TECHNIQUE
Axial view of the calcaneus.

CALCANEUS SECUNDARIUS
Rare accessory ossicle—sometimes fused to the calcaneus giving a spur appearance. It occurs as a small, irregular, quadrilateral bone lying in the angle between the calcaneus, astragalus, cuboid, and navicular.
TECHNIQUE
Lateral tarsus.

CALCAREOUS TENDINITIS
Calcification in the tendon-sheaths. The most common site for the condition is near the insertion of the supraspinatus tendon into the greater tuberosity of the humerus, but it may also occur at the insertion of the infraspinatus or biceps tendon. It is more common in patients of middle age.
TECHNIQUE
AP shoulder, as routine.
1. **Supraspinatus**
   AP shoulder with arm internally rotated and adducted—10 kV less to show soft tissue.
2. **Infraspinatus**
   AP shoulder with hand pronated to side of the body with thumb forward to show calcification in profile.
3. **Biceps**
   Bicipital groove—for long head of biceps (*see* APPENDIX).

CALCIFIED ABDOMINAL AORTA

Calcification of the aorta, almost always associated with atheromatous degeneration.

TECHNIQUE

Lateral abdomen.

CALCIFIED ABDOMINAL GLANDS

Usually presumed to be of tuberculous origin, occurring mainly in the mesenteric glands. Shadows are granular and mottled.

TECHNIQUE

AP abdomen.

Lateral abdomen.

CALCIFIED CHOROID PLEXUS

Calcification may occur in the choroid plexuses of the lateral ventricles. The radiographic appearance is that of a small number of calcified points gathered together, and of less density than pineal calcifications. It is usually bilateral lying approximately 2 cm behind and below the pineal shadow.

TECHNIQUE

PA skull.

Lateral skull.

Towne's view.

CALCIFIED GALL-BLADDER (Porcelain Gall-bladder)

The wall of the gall-bladder is calcified, a rare occurrence, occurring only with pre-existing fibrosis. Calcium is laid down symmetrically and ovoid outline of the gall-bladder is demonstrated.

TECHNIQUE

PA right hypochondrium.

Right lateral hypochondrium.

CALCIFIED PINEAL BODY

Calcification laid down in the central part of the body usually with advancing age. Calcification alone is of little significance, but the fact that the pineal is demonstrated is an aid to diagnosis in space-occupying lesions.

TECHNIQUE

AP skull with 35° caudal tilt.

Lateral skull.

CALCIFIED SUPRASPINATUS

See CALCAREOUS TENDINITIS.

CALCINOSIS CIRCUMSCRIPTA (Hypodermolithiasis)

Calcified nodules limited to the skin and subcutaneous tissues of the upper extremities, particularly the hands.

TECHNIQUE

PA hands.

CALCINOSIS UNIVERSALIS

Calcified nodules which are widespread and involve muscles, tendons, and nerve-sheaths, as well as subcutaneous tissues. It is more frequently seen in children, calcified masses often occurring in the region of the larger joints.

TECHNIQUE

AP affected area.

Lateral affected area.

CARCINOMATOSIS

Widespread dissemination of malignant deposits occurring in many organs as well as frequently in the bones. Those normally involved in the latter are the skull, spine, pelvis, and upper ends of the femur, humerus, and ribs.

TECHNIQUE

AP affected area.

Lateral affected area.

A skeletal survey may be required—*see* APPENDIX.

CARDIAC ANEURYSM

A localized bulging of the heart occurring as a late complication of a coronary thrombosis and myocardial infarction.

TECHNIQUE

PA chest.

Penetrated PA chest—increase 10 kV.

Right and left anterior oblique.

CARDIAC HYPERTROPHY

See HEART, ENLARGEMENT OF.

CARDIOSPASM

See ACHALASIA OF THE CARDIA.

CARPAL TUNNEL SYNDROME

A symptom complex due to the compression of the median nerve within the carpal tunnel.

TECHNIQUE
PA wrist.
Lateral wrist.
Carpal tunnel view—*see* APPENDIX.

CERVICAL RIB

Rudimentary or well-formed rib arising from the 7th
cervical vertebra causing pressure on the brachial
plexus; although rare, ribs may also arise from the
5th and 6th cervical vertebrae.
TECHNIQUE
AP cervico-dorsal spine.

CHARCOT'S JOINT

Neurogenic arthropathy often associated with tabes
dorsalis and syringomyelia. Any joint may be
affected, but most common sites are the knee,
ankle, and foot. In the later stages there is loss of
joint space, increase in bone density, and disorgani-
zation of the joint.
TECHNIQUE
AP affected area.
Lateral affected area.
Increase in penetration is necessary if the disease is
of long standing.

CHLOROMA

Multiple tumours of the bones, viscera, and lymph-
nodes. Clinically the disease resembles leukaemia
and is more frequently seen in children than in
adults. The usual site is the skull, but the spine,
ribs, sternum, pelvis, and long bones may also be
affected. Bone destruction is seen as 'punched-out'
areas and may be visible around the tumour.
TECHNIQUE
AP skull.
Lateral skull.

CHOLECYSTOGASTRIC FISTULA

A track uniting the stomach and the gall-bladder
resulting from perforation of a gastric ulcer or
ulceration of a gall-stone through the gall-bladder
wall.
TECHNIQUE
Erect AP abdomen—to show air track.

CHOLELITHIASIS
Gall-stones formed as a result of precipitation of bile-salts.
TECHNIQUE
PA right hypochondrium.
Lateral right hypochondrium.
Ultrasound.

CHOLESTEATOMA (Pearly Tumour)
A result of chronic infection in the middle ear consisting of an overgrowth of epithelium and sometimes containing cholesterol.
TECHNIQUE
35° fronto-occipital.
Right and left lateral obliques of mastoids—pinna of the ear forward.

CHONDROCALCINOSIS (Pseudo-gout)
Characterized by the presence of calcium pyrophosphate crystals in the synovial fluid, and accompanied by attacks of joint pain. Fibrocartilaginous or hyaline cartilage calcification suggests this diagnosis. In an acute attack there is often evidence of joint effusion. The most common site is the knee involving the menisci. Diagnosis is strengthened by calcification of the symphysis pubis and calcification in other joints.
TECHNIQUE
AP both knees.
AP symphysis pubis.

CHONDROMA
A benign tumour arising from cartilage. Radiologically the tumour produces a rarefaction when the affected part of the bone is centrally situated. If, however, it is in the cortex this may present an area of erosion, with a faint shadow projecting into the soft tissue. A single chondroma is comparatively rare, but may occur in the phalanges.
TECHNIQUE
PA hands.
AP and lateral affected area.

CHONDROMALACIA PATELLAE
A degenerative change in the cartilage of the patella, occasionally visible as an area of subarticular translucency.

TECHNIQUE
PA knee.
Lateral knee.
Skyline view of both patellae.
AP tomograms—if required.

CHORDOMA

A locally malignant tumour derived from remnants of the notochord, commonest in the sacrum and upper cervical area.

TECHNIQUE
AP pelvis.
Lateral cervical spine.

CHROMOPHOBE ADENOMA

A tumour arising in the anterior lobe of the pituitary gland, often causing radiological changes in the appearance of the sella turcica.

TECHNIQUE
AP skull with 35° caudal tilt (Towne's view).
Lateral skull.

CLEIDO-CRANIAL DYOSTOSIS

A congenital deformity resulting in incomplete ossification of the skull, and deformities or absence of the clavicles. There may be associated deformities in other parts of the skeleton.

TECHNIQUE
AP pelvis—to show widened symphysis pubis.
PA skull.
Lateral skull.
AP both shoulders and clavicles on one film.
Upper and lower jaws—for dental eruption.

CLUB FOOT

See TALIPES EQUINOVARUS.

COARCTATION OF THE AORTA

Congenital stenosis of the distal part of the aortic arch. Compensatory collateral circulation develops in the arteries arising proximal to the segment, giving characteristic rib notching (Roestler's sign).

TECHNIQUE
PA chest.
Right anterior oblique.
Left lateral.
AP chest with 5° cephalic tilt—for early diagnosis.

COELIAC DISEASE
See STEATORRHOEA.

COLD ABSCESS
A tuberculous abscess in the soft tissues. It follows the fascial planes and appears in the paraspinal region or along the sheath of the psoas.
TECHNIQUE
See PARAVERTEBRAL ABSCESS or PSOAS ABSCESS.

CONGENITAL DISLOCATION OF THE HIP (CDH)
See DISLOCATION OF THE HIP, CONGENITAL.

CONRADI'S DISEASE
See DYSPLASIA EPIPHYSIALIS CALCIFICANS.

COOLEY'S ANAEMIA
See THALASSAEMIA.

CORONARY THROMBOSIS
A clot of blood forming in the arterial circulation. This is almost always associated with atheroma and results in death of the heart muscle supplied by that artery with consequent infarction and eventual fibrosis.
TECHNIQUE
PA chest—for heart size, and for coronary artery calcification.

COR PULMONALE
A disease of the heart due to the obstruction of the pulmonary circulation. The increase in the load is on the right side of the heart producing right ventricular failure.
TECHNIQUE
PA chest at 2 m.
Lateral chest.
Left anterior oblique.

COXA VARA
A condition in which the neck of the femur is bent downwards. This may reach such an extent that the neck forms a right-angle or less with the shaft of the femur, the usual angle being $120-140°$. This condition usually results from a slipped epiphysis, but it can be tuberculous or congenital in origin, and in its most severe form is associated with absence of the proximal portion of the femur.

TECHNIQUE

AP pelvis—to show both hip-joints. (The feet of the patient must be perpendicular to the table and symmetrical.)

CRANIOPHARYNGIOMA (Rathke's Pouch Tumour)

A rare tumour of the Rathke pouch, which is a remnant of fetal life, arising from the nasopharynx. The pituitary fossa may enlarge, and frequently the tumour calcifies.

TECHNIQUE

Lateral coned pituitary fossa.
Lateral skull.
PA skull.
AP skull with 30° caudal tilt.
Submento-vertical.
Soft-tissue lateral may be required to see minute calcification.

CRANIOSTENOSIS

The premature closing of one or more cranial sutures, resulting in a small skull. This term embraces various skull deformities which arise from the above cause, and includes oxycephaly, scaphocephaly, craniofacial dysostosis, and plagiocephaly. This condition is thought to be a congenital abnormality.

TECHNIQUE

PA skull.
Lateral skull.

CRANIOTABES

A condition occurring in infancy. It is the formation of conical areas in bone substance which are small and shallow, mainly in the frontal and parietal bones of the skull. It usually results from rickets, narasmus or syphilis.

TECHNIQUE

PA skull.
Lateral skull.

CRETINISM

A congenital thyroid deficiency, resulting in very slow growth often associated with mental retardation. The bones are thick and short, the epiphyses appear late and are often irregular and deformed. The fontanelles remain open and dentition is delayed.

TECHNIQUE

PA skull.

Lateral skull.

PA wrist and hand—for assessment of skeletal age.

AP pelvis—to show possible fragmented capital epiphysis.

CROHN'S DISEASE

A chronic, non-specific, granulomatous process, frequently involving the terminal portion of the ileum. It may also extend to the large colon or arise in the proximal ileum.

TECHNIQUE

Demonstrated only by the use of opaque media. When radiological advice is not available, barium can be given to drink and films taken in the supine position at hourly intervals from 4 to 8 hours, and a final film at 24 hours.

CUSHING'S SYNDROME

The loss of granules in the basophil cells of the pituitary gland, being more common in women. There is persistent hypertension, and generalized osteoporosis may occur, resulting in spontaneous fractures.

TECHNIQUE

AP skull with $35°$ caudal tilt.

Lateral skull.

PA chest—to demonstrate rib fractures.

(In a child views for skeletal maturity may be required.)

Lateral dorsal and lumbar spine—to demonstrate any osteoporosis.

CYSTADENOMA

An ovarian neoplasm which may attain tremendous size, producing a soft-tissue swelling, and causing elevation of the diaphragm and visceral displacement.

TECHNIQUE

PA abdomen—erect to include diaphragm.

CYSTICERCOSIS

An infestation by parasites known as cysticerci, which are the larval stage of the tapeworm. It only becomes radiologically important when these parasites become calcified. The areas most commonly affected are the muscles of the lower leg and thigh, and the brain.

TECHNIQUE

Lateral skull.

AP femur—to include hip-joint.

Lateral tibia and fibula—to include knee-joint.

As these demonstrate as soft-tissue opacities, a reduction of mA.s. is recommended.

CYSTOLITHS

Stones in the bladder which can grow to a considerable size.

TECHNIQUE

AP bladder with $15°$ caudal tilt.

DACTYLITIS

An inflammation of the fingers and toes. It may be tuberculous, when it is referred to as spina ventosa, or it may be caused by syphilis, leprosy, or yaws, the radiological appearance varying according to type.

TECHNIQUE

PA hands.

AP feet.

DECOMPRESSION SICKNESS

See CAISSON DISEASE.

DIAPHYSEAL ACLASIS

Exostosis from the diaphysis of the bones, which may cause pressure symptoms. Apart from the exostosis there is often a marked deformity of the forearm, where the ulna is found to be short and the distal epiphysis defective. The most common sites for exostoses are the shafts of long bones and the pelvis.

TECHNIQUE

AP forearms.

AP long bones.

AP pelvis.

DIAPHYSEAL DYSPLASIA (Engelmann's Disease)

A benign bone disease characterized by symmetrical fusiform enlargement and sclerosis of the long bones—often associated with changes in the skull.

TECHNIQUE

AP and lateral affected area.

AP and lateral skull.

DIASTASIS OF THE SYMPHYSIS PUBIS

There may be a widening of this joint in early pregnancy or during prolonged labour. The separation is horizontal, but may also be vertical when the patient is weight bearing. This examination should not be done during pregnancy owing to the risk of genetic dangers.

TECHNIQUE

PA symphysis pubis—prone.

PA symphysis pubis—erect, weight bearing on the right foot.

PA symphysis pubis—weight bearing on the left foot.

DIETL'S CRISIS

A severe nephralgia, chills and vomiting and general collapse, resulting from angulation of a ureter caused by a floating kidney.

TECHNIQUE

AP abdomen—for urinary tract.

Erect AP abdomen—to demonstrate displacement of kidney.

DISLOCATION OF HIP—CONGENITAL (CDH)

A congenital deformity where there is either complete dislocation or only subluxation of the hip. It may be unilateral or bilateral, the former being more common. It is more easily recognized after the appearance of the epiphysis of the femoral head which is usually smaller than normal and misaligned. Before the epiphyseal appearance the signs are only obvious from the defective development of the acetabulum.

TECHNIQUE

AP pelvis—feet in the neutral position.

AP pelvis—von Rosen's projection—this view can produce false negatives and positives and should only be used with medical supervision—*see* APPENDIX.

DISLOCATION OF THE PATELLA—RECURRENT

A slipping of the patella over the lateral condyle of the femur which is flattened, causing a shallow intercondylar groove. Frequent dislocations produce osteochondritis and loose bodies, and roughening of the medial side of the patella.

TECHNIQUE
    PA knee.
    Lateral knee.
    Skyline view of patellae with knees flexed at $35°$, tube horizontal, film at right-angles to the tube.
    Intercondylar view both knees.

DISLOCATION OF THE SHOULDER

1. **Anterior.** Most common type.
   TECHNIQUE
       AP shoulder.
       Lateral shoulder—through the body.
2. **Recurrent.** With this type of dislocation there is often a 'hatchet defect' on the humeral head. The original dislocation is usually due to trauma.
   TECHNIQUE
       AP shoulder with $30°$ abduction and $45°$ internal rotation of the humerus, combined with $15°$ caudal tube tilt.
       Axial view.
       Stryker's projection—*see* APPENDIX.
3. **Posterior.** Resulting from trauma. This condition is more difficult to diagnose clinically and radiologically than the more common anterior dislocation.
   TECHNIQUE
       AP shoulder.
       Infero-superior axial view.

DISLOCATION OF THE TALUS AND/OR CUBOID

Injury to tarsus due to severe trauma.
TECHNIQUE
    AP foot with $5-10°$ cephalic tilt to separate tarsal bones.
    Dorsiplantar oblique.
    True lateral.

DISSECTING ANEURYSM

The result of blood entering into the wall of an artery (usually the ascending aorta) and tracking upwards and downwards between the layers of the vessel wall. It may eventually rupture outwards at a point some distance from the internal entry point.
TECHNIQUE
    PA chest.
    Lateral chest.
    Right and left anterior obliques.

DOWN'S SYNDROME
See MONGOLISM.

DRACUNCULUS MEDINENSIS
Infestation by the guinea worm—not unlike cysticer-
cosis except that the parasite is much longer, and
the appearance when calcified shows more elonga-
ted areas of calcification. The areas most commonly
affected are the subcutaneous tissues of the foot
and lower leg.
TECHNIQUE
Lateral foot and leg—reduce mA.s. to show soft
tissue.

DRILLER'S DISEASE (Vibration Syndrome)
Degenerative cystic changes in the wrist and hand
develop as a result of prolonged use of vibrating
tools, often more marked in the guiding hand.
TECHNIQUE
PA both hands and wrists.

DUODENAL ATRESIA
A complete or partial obstruction of the duodenum
by a transverse membrane, usually between the 1st
and 2nd part of the duodenum with no gas in
distal part of the gut.
TECHNIQUE
1. **Supine Abdomen.** Care must be taken to ensure
the patient is in the true AP position to demonstrate the 'double bubble' appearance of air in the
stomach and 1st part of the duodenum.
2. **Erect Abdomen.** This may be needed for differential diagnosis and for confirmation of position of
the gas shadows.

DWARFISM
An abnormal underdevelopment of the body. There
are several types but in all of them deficient cal-
cium in the bones is usually radiologically apparent.
TECHNIQUE
PA wrists.
AP ankles and knees.
Lateral skull for pituitary fossa.

DYSCHONDROPLASIA
A congenital abnormality resulting from partial
failure of ossification of the metaphysial cartilage.

Translucent columns of cartilage are shown in the shafts of the long bones.

TECHNIQUE

AP pelvis.

AP long bones.

DYSPLASIA EPIPHYSIALIS CALCIFICANS (Conradi's Disease)

The abnormalities of this disease are not confined to the skeletal system but radiological appearances may overshadow extra-skeletal features. The radiological appearances consist of dense and stippled calcifications within the cartilaginous parts of every bone undergoing enchondral ossification. These changes are prominent in the region of the epiphyses of the long bones especially hips and shoulders but they may also occur in the carpus and tarsus, in the spine and in the tracheal and laryngeal cartilages.

TECHNIQUE

AP both hips.

AP both shoulders.

Lateral spine.

AP feet.

PA wrists.

DYSPLASIA EPIPHYSIALIS MULTIPLEX

A familial condition primarily affecting the epiphyses. These tend to be flattened and fragmented and appear late. These deformities are permanent.

TECHNIQUE

AP hips.

AP and lateral knees.

AP shoulders.

AP and lateral elbows.

Hands, wrists and feet.

EBSTEIN'S DISEASE

A rare condition of the tricuspid valve in which there are various abnormalities, the most important of which is that the posterior cusp is not attached to the annulus.

TECHNIQUE

PA chest, fairly penetrated—to show enlargement of the right ventricle.

ECHINOCOCCOSIS

Infestation by small tapeworm in its larval or hydatid stage——the most common site being the liver, and secondly the lungs.

TECHNIQUE

See HYDATID DISEASE.

ECTOPIA VESICAE

Developmental failure in the bladder and genital organs. The symphysis pubis is underdeveloped.

TECHNIQUE

AP bladder——to include symphysis pubis.

ECTOPIC LUNG SEGMENT

An extra lung segment supplied by an aberrant artery.

TECHNIQUE

PA chest.

Lateral chest.

Tomography——if required.

EMPYEMA

The presence of pus within a hollow organ or cavity.

TECHNIQUE

Any projection required to demonstrate this condition should be taken in the erect or decubitus position.

ENCHONDROMATA

Benign tumours of cartilage which grow within the interior of the bone, the most common site being that of the hands, where they produce a bubble-like appearance radiologically.

TECHNIQUE

AP affected area.

Lateral affected area.

PA both hands.

ENCRUSTED CYSTITIS

Small calcified deposits giving diffuse mottling of the bladder.

TECHNIQUE

AP bladder with 15° caudal tilt.

ENDOCARDITIS

A disease of the inner heart-lining by bacterial or viral infection. The organisms travel in the blood-stream and set up distant foci of infection or grow on the heart-valves causing scarring and deformity.

TECHNIQUE
PA chest at 2 m—for heart size.

ENGELMANN'S DISEASE
See DIAPHYSEAL DYSPLASIA.

EOSINOPHIL ADENOMA
See ACROMEGALY and GIGANTISM.

EOSINOPHIL GRANULOMA
See HAND–SCHÜLLER–CHRISTIAN DISEASE.

EPIDEMIC PLEURODYNIA (Bornholm's Disease)
A syndrome of unknown origin, characterized by sudden onset of severe pain in the abdominal wall and intercostal spaces. It is usually accompanied by a mild fever.
TECHNIQUE
PA chest.

ERYTHEMA NODOSUM
A disease which is often an allergic response to certain drugs, tubercular or streptococcal infection, and sarcoidosis. There are thickened reddish areas on the skin of the shins, forearms, and hands.
TECHNIQUE
PA chest—for tuberculosis and hilar enlargement.
PA hands.

EWING'S TUMOUR
A rare malignant tumour of bone, most commonly found in the centre of the shaft of long bones and ribs. Children and young adults are affected.
TECHNIQUE
AP affected area.
Lateral affected area.

EXOPHTHALMIC GOITRE (Graves' Disease)
A diffuse goitre with hyperthyroidism occurring in young and middle-aged adults. There is an increase in the metabolic rate, nervous excitability, and tachycardia. Cardiac damage frequently occurs.
TECHNIQUE
PA chest—to include thoracic inlet.
Lateral thoracic inlet. (Flying angel technique—*see* APPENDIX.)
Lateral skull—for pituitary fossa.

FABELLA

Small, rounded sesamoid bone found in the tendon of the lateral head of the gastrocnemius, in the posterior part of the leg near the knee-joint. It is seen to lie on the lateral side of the knee in the AP view.

TECHNIQUE

AP knee-joint.

Lateral knee-joint.

FAIRBANK'S SHELF OPERATION

This is the creating of a false acetabulum with a shelf of bone placed superiorly.

TECHNIQUE

AP hip-joint.

FALLOT'S TETRALOGY

Consists of a group of four conditions:

1. Pulmonary stenosis.
2. Defective intraventricular septum.
3. Dextra position of the aorta.
4. Hypertrophy of right ventricle.

This causes cyanosis and shortness of breath. Radiologically some 50 per cent of cases show a 'boot-shaped' heart and a deficiency in vascular markings.

TECHNIQUE

PA chest at 2 m—for heart size.

Left anterior oblique.

In the neonate—AP chest supine (to reduce likelihood of cardiac arrest).

FANCONI SYNDROME

A form of rickets associated with renal disease.

TECHNIQUE

See RICKETS.

FETAL DEATH IN UTERO

The possible indications are overlap of the cranial bones (Spalding's sign), air in the great vessels (Rowan Williams's sign), or hyperflexion.

TECHNIQUE

Ultrasound.

PA abdomen prone for confirmation.

FETAL PRESENTATION IN UTERO

Three main types of presentation are recognized—breach, vertex, and transverse.

TECHNIQUE
AP abdomen.
(The mother should take a few deep breaths prior
to exposure, to prevent fetal movement caused
by anoxaemia. Careful compression can also
be made by the use of a broad compression
band.)

FIBROCYSTIC DISEASE OF THE PANCREAS
An obstructive disease of the mucous glands of the
pancreas occurring simultaneously in the glands of
the bronchi and intestines. It is most common in
infants under 1 year old and often results in early
death from respiratory infection.
TECHNIQUE
AP abdomen.
PA chest.

FILARIA BANCROFTI
Worm infestation causing lymphatic obstruction,
which when calcified often appears in the soft tissue
of the leg or thigh. As calcified and live worms
are found in the same region, the areas to be
examined should be those of maximum tenderness.
TECHNIQUE
AP pelvic area—to include genitalia.
AP and lateral affected area.

FLAT FOOT
See TALIPES PLANUS.

FLUOROSIS
Poisoning by absorption of toxic amounts of fluoride.
Radiologically this shows as an increase in skeletal
density. Bony growths may appear where ligaments
are attached, most commonly seen in the pelvis,
forearm, and lower leg. There may also be con-
siderable lipping of the vertebral bodies, especially
lumbar.
TECHNIQUE
AP pelvis.
AP forearm and lower leg.
Lateral lumbar spine.

FONG'S DISEASE (Nail Patella Syndrome)

A congenital skeletal deformity where there is an absence of patellae, dystrophy of the nails and hypoplasia of the capitellum and radial head. There may also be bony horns protruding dorsally from the ilium.

TECHNIQUE
   Lateral knees.
   AP pelvis.
   AP and lateral elbows.

FRAGILITAS OSSIUM

See OSTEOGENESIS IMPERFECTA.

FREIBERG'S DISEASE

Osteochondritis of the metatarsal heads, usually second or third.

TECHNIQUE
   AP both feet.
   Dorsiplantar oblique both feet.

FRIEDRICH'S ATAXIA

An hereditary disease with a lateral curvature of the spine and spinal sclerosis. There is lower limb palsy and impairment of speech.

TECHNIQUE
   Films to demonstrate scoliosis and kypho-scoliosis due to progressive muscular weakness.
   Chest—to demonstrate myocardiopathy.

FROSTBITE (In children)

No immediate sign but mild osteoporosis may occur 1 to 2 months later. In some cases however punched out per-articular defects may appear between 6 to 10 months. Severe frostbite can cause injury to the epiphyses and then the cartilages, leading later to deformity and shortening of digits involved.

TECHNIQUE
   PA hands.
   AP feet.

FROZEN SHOULDER

The clinical diagnosis of a condition whereby there is gross limitation of movement in all directions accompanied by pain. Calcification may be shown in the supraspinatus tendon-sheath.

TECHNIQUE
AP shoulder with internal and external rotation.
Axial view.

FUNNEL CHEST
A depression of the lower third of the sternum causing abnormal heart-sounds and heart outline. It is congenital in origin and may be associated with congenital heart disease.
TECHNIQUE
PA chest.
Left lateral chest——in cases with no heart shadow to the right of the spine.
Lateral on inspiration and expiration——for range of movement.

GALEAZZI FRACTURE
A fracture of the radius with overlap of the fragments and dislocation of the head of the ulna.
TECHNIQUE
AP   }   Whole length of the forearm——to include both the wrist and elbow-joint.
Lateral }

GARDNER'S SYNDROME
A familial cutaneous disease the salient features of which are multiple colonic polyps, multiple osteomas especially on the facial bones, in particular the mandible and the maxilla, and also the skull. There may also be cortical thickening of the diaphyses of one or more of the long bones.
TECHNIQUE
PA mandible.
Occipito-mental view with 30° caudal tilt.
AP and lateral of the affected long bones.

GAS GANGRENE
A systemic infection by gas-forming bacteria. It may be caused by soft-tissue trauma, abortion, or by faecal contamination entering the blood from a bowel cancer.
TECHNIQUE
AP affected area.
Lateral affected area, with horizontal beam to demonstrate air in the tissue.

GAUCHER'S DISEASE

A disease of the reticulo-endothelial system, the cells containing large amounts of kerasin, causing enlargement of the spleen. Radiologically the affected bones show diffuse or patchy osteoporosis and thinning of the cortex, which may in some cases become expanded. Widening of the lower ends of the femora is characteristic of this disease due to the disturbance in enchondral ossification.

TECHNIQUE
AP affected area.
Lateral affected area.
AP lower ends of femur.

GEE'S DISEASE

See STEATORRHOEA, IDIOPATHIC.

GENU VALGUM

A condition of inward curving of the knee—this can be unilateral or bilateral and is commonly known as 'knock-knees'.

TECHNIQUE
Long leg film-erect to include ankle and hip joints for accurate assessment of the angles of surgical correction.

GENU VARUM

A condition of outward bowing of the leg—commonly known as 'bow-legs'.

TECHNIQUE
As above.

GHON FOCUS

Primary pulmonary tuberculous lesion.

TECHNIQUE
PA chest.

GIANT-CELL TUMOUR

The majority of these tumours are thought to be benign, although they may have malignant tendencies. These lesions are usually found in the ends of the long bones, the knee being the most common site.

TECHNIQUE
AP affected area.
Lateral affected area.

GIGANTISM

Excess of growth hormone of the anterior pituitary gland before the fusion of the epiphysis.

TECHNIQUE

Lateral pituitary fossa.
PA hand and wrist—for bone age.
Unilateral skeletal survey.

GLANDULAR FEVER

A virus infection causing fever and glandular enlargement with abnormal cells and lymphocytes in the blood-stream.

TECHNIQUE

PA chest—for enlarged hilar glands.

GLOMUS JUGULAR TUMOUR

A tumour arising from small masses of epithelioid tissue in the region of the jugular bulb. It may invade the petrous bone and floor of the posterior fossa.

TECHNIQUE

PA skull with 10° caudal tilt.
AP skull with 35° caudal tilt (Towne's view).
Right and left lateral skull.
Submento-vertical.
Tomography.

GOUT

A metabolic disturbance where the small joint symptoms are dominant—most frequently those of the hands and feet.

TECHNIQUE

PA hands.
AP feet.

GRAVES' DISEASE

See EXOPHTHALMIC GOITRE.

GREIG'S DISEASE

See HYPERTELORISM.

HAEMANGIOMA

A benign tumour composed of blood-vessels which may be found in the bones or soft tissue. Calcified bodies resembling pheboliths may be seen in the area. Where there is bone involvement, the most common site is the spine.

TECHNIQUE
AP affected area.
Lateral affected area.

HAEMARTHROSES
Haemorrhages into joints—common in haemophilia. Severe arthritic changes may occur with repeated haemorrhages which will eventually lead to ankylosis.
TECHNIQUE
AP affected joint.
Lateral affected joint—with horizontal beam.
Tunnel view on relevant joint—to demonstrate characteristic widening of the notch occurring in haemophilia.

HALLUX RIGIDUS
A restricted range of movements in the first metatarso-phalangeal joint, frequently secondary to degenerative joint disease.
TECHNIQUE
AP feet.
Lateral feet—to show presence of osteophytes on the dorsum of the joint.

HALLUX VALGUS
The deviation of the first metatarsal from the second metatarsal, with the phalanges bent towards the second toe causing prominence of the metatarso-phalangeal joint.
TECHNIQUE
AP feet.

HAND—SCHÜLLER—CHRISTIAN DISEASE
An osseous type of histiocytosis. A disease of the reticulo-endothelial system. Usually affects older children and adults. There is an abnormal accumulation of lipoids in the reticulo-endothelial system, and multiple areas of bone destruction occur mainly in the flat bones, especially in the skull where it may present a 'map-like' appearance. Closely related to the above condition are eosinophil granuloma and Letterer-Siwe disease.

TECHNIQUE
Lateral skull.
PA chest—for lung involvement and pathological fractures of ribs.
AP pelvis.

HATCHET DEFECT OF THE SHOULDER
See DISLOCATION OF THE SHOULDER—RECURRENT.

HEART, ENLARGEMENT OF (Cardiac Hypertrophy)
There are many causes for enlargement of the heart including valvular diseases, endocrine disturbances, and hypertension, etc.
TECHNIQUE
PA chest at 2 m—for heart size.
Right and left anterior oblique.
Left lateral chest.

HEBERDEN'S NODES
Degenerative arthritis producing nodular enlargement around the terminal joints of the fingers.
TECHNIQUE
PA hands.

HIATUS HERNIA
The fundus of the stomach penetrates the oesophageal hiatus of the diaphragm into the thoracic cavity. Gas and fluid levels may be seen through the heart shadow.
TECHNIQUE
PA chest—penetrated ⎞
Lateral chest ⎠ Erect.

HILAR LYMPH-GLANDS, ENLARGEMENT OF
The enlargement of these nodes occurs in various diseases involving the lymph-glands, such as Hodgkin's disease, lymphosarcoma, and sarcoidosis, and is occasionally the sequel to some lung diseases.
TECHNIQUE
PA chest.
Left anterior oblique—to bring tracheal bifurcation into relief to show proximal lymph-nodes.
Left lateral chest.

HIRSCHSPRUNG'S DISEASE

Great dilatation of the colon, mainly the distal portions. It is usually congenital, although often only discovered in adult life. In some cases the enormous dilatation of the splenic flexure may cause the diaphragm to be pushed upwards causing dyspnoea.

TECHNIQUE

AP abdomen.

AP abdomen erect—to include diaphragm.

N.B. This disease is diagnosed by rectal biopsy and the extent demonstrated by barium enema.

HODGKIN'S DISEASE

This disease is generally considered to be a form of cancer involving the reticulo-endothelial system, notably the lymph-glands with resultant enlargement.

TECHNIQUE

PA chest.

AP abdomen—to demonstrate spleen.

HORNER'S SYNDROME

Unilateral ptosis, miosis, enopthalmos, reduced sweating, and flushing of the face due to destruction of the cervical sympathetic system of the same side.

TECHNIQUE

PA chest.

AP and lateral of the cervical spine.

HORSESHOE KIDNEY

A developmental anomaly whereby both kidneys are joined by an isthmus of renal tissue, usually at the lower poles. The kidneys are always in an unusually low position in this condition and may be turned around with the ureters placed laterally.

TECHNIQUE

AP abdomen on inspiration and expiration—to show mobility and outline.

HOUR-GLASS TUMOUR

See NEUROFIBROMA.

HUNTER'S SYNDROME

See also MUCOPOLYSACCHARIDOSES.

This is an X-linked recessive form of mucopolysaccharidoses which can vary in severity combined with various degrees of mental retardation. These skeletal changes can include microcephaly, J-shaped sella turcica, thickened calvaria, oar-shaped ribs, hook-shaped vertebral bodies and changes in the pelvis.

TECHNIQUE
Lateral skull.
AP ribs.
Lateral vertebral bodies.
AP pelvis.

HURLER'S DISEASE (*See* MUCOPOLYSACCHARIDOSES)

A congenital disease characterized by dwarfism, with short kyphotic spinal column, short fingers, depression of the bridge of the nose, grotesquely large head, hepatosplenomegaly and mental deficiency.

TECHNIQUE
Lateral lumbar spine—to differentiate from Morquio—Brailsford disease.
Lateral skull—to show sella turcica which may become J-shaped.
PA hands.
AP pelvis—to demonstrate possible coxa valga deformity.
Lateral spine.

HYDATID DISEASE OF THE LIVER

An infection due to tapeworm. Cysts form and calcification of the cyst wall is frequent.

TECHNIQUE
Where ultrasound is not available.
AP upper abdomen.
Lateral upper abdomen.
PA chest ⎫ Similar infection can be trans-
Lateral chest ⎰ mitted to lung and other areas.

HYDRAMNION

Excessive amniotic fluid, a condition which is frequently associated with multiple pregnancy or fetal abnormality.

TECHNIQUE
Ultrasound.
In the case of fetal abnormality, ultrasound is used for the primary diagnosis.
For confirmation
PA abdomen ⎫ with increased penetration.
Lateral abdomen ⎰

HYDROCEPHALUS

An excessive accumulation of cerebrospinal fluid within the cranium, causing gross enlargement and thinning of the vault of the skull with enlarged fontanelles.

TECHNIQUE

In utero

Ultrasound.

In child

Ultrasound if fontanelles are still open.

AP skull.

Lateral skull.

HYDROPNEUMOTHORAX

A mixture of air and fluid present in the pleural cavity.

TECHNIQUE

PA chest ⎫ Erect, centring through the fluid
Lateral chest ⎬ level to define.

HYDROPS FETALIS

Changes in the fetus caused by haemolysis. These changes produce a 'halo' shadow around the fetal skull, and the fetus lies in the 'Buddha' position.

TECHNIQUE

Ultrasound is used for primary diagnosis followed by

PA abdomen ⎫ for confirmation.
Lateral abdomen ⎬

HYPERCALCAEMIA

An excessive quantity of calcium contained in the blood.

TECHNIQUE

PA hands.

AP feet.

Lateral skull.

AP abdomen—to demonstrate nephrocalcinosis.

HYPERFLEXION SIGN

The fetus lies in an exaggerated attitude as if rolled into a ball. This is suggestive of fetal death.

TECHNIQUE

Ultrasound is used for primary diagnosis followed by

PA abdomen ⎫ for confirmation.
Lateral abdomen ⎬

HYPEROSTOSIS CRANII

An increase in bone mass usually due to the invasion by a bone tumour. It can also be due to inflammation or endocrine disturbance.

TECHNIQUE

AP skull with 35° caudal tilt.

PA skull with 20° caudal tilt.

Lateral skull.

Tangential views.

HYPERPARATHYROIDISM (Osteitis Fibrosa Cystica)

Overactivity of the parathyroid glands which control the amounts of calcium phosphate in the blood. There may be cardiac enlargement and calcifica-cation, an excess of calcium excreted in the urine, and the bones may become osteoporotic. The skull becomes thickened and presents a mottled appearance with less definite inner and outer table contours.

TECHNIQUE

PA skull.

Lateral skull.

PA chest.

Hands, clavicles, humeri, radii, and ulnae——affected towards their extremities.

HYPERTELORISM (Greig's Disease)

A deformity of the frontal region of the cranium resembling mongolism and associated with mental deficiency. It also shows abnormal growth of the cartilaginous base of the skull, and radiologically enlarged lesser wings and diminished greater wings of the sphenoid are demonstrated.

TECHNIQUE

PA skull with 10° caudal tilt.

Lateral skull.

Submento-vertical.

HYPERTENSION

This is a condition of raised blood-pressure either as a result of small artery contraction and spasm, or secondary to disease elsewhere.

TECHNIQUE

PA chest.

HYPERTENSIVE HEART DISEASE

To sustain a high blood-pressure, extra work load is required by the left ventricle which hypertrophies as a result. In this disease the heart is enlarged and eventually causes heart failure.

TECHNIQUE

PA chest at 2 m—for heart size.

HYPODERMOLITHIASIS

See CALCINOSIS CIRCUMSCRIPTA.

HYPOTHYROIDISM

See CRETINISM.

IMPERFORATE ANUS

This term includes both high and low atresias of the gut of which there are a number of variants and there is no ideal single classification. Where plain radiography is requested the neonate should be at least 18 hours old.

TECHNIQUE

Invert the child for 5—15 minutes to allow rectal gas to rise to demonstrate position of septum. Place blob of thick barium at skin surface approximate to anal orifice.

Lateral rectum centred on the greater trochanter with patient inverted.

AP supine film.

(There are often associated abnormalities).

INFANTILE CORTICAL HYPEROSTOSIS

See CAFFEY'S DISEASE.

INFERTILITY

Infertility can be caused by the toxic effect of tubercular infection, or by a tumour or mass situated proximally to the pituitary fossa.

TECHNIQUE

PA chest.

Lateral pituitary fossa.

Towne's view—to project the pituitary fossa in the foramen magnum.

AP pelvis—for calcification.

INFRASPINATUS CALCIFICATION

See CALCAREOUS TENDINITIS.

INTERMITTENT CLAUDICATION

Weakness and cramp in the legs, more especially the calves, induced by exertion and relieved by rest, associated with peripheral vascular disease which results from extensive atheroma.

TECHNIQUE

Lateral femora   } For atheromatous
Lateral tibiae and fibulae   }   calcification.
PA chest.

INTESTINAL OBSTRUCTION, ACUTE

The prevention of the normal passage of faeces and flatus, which may be partial or complete. It can be caused by a volvulus, intussusception, etc., or changes in the bowel wall as in carcinoma, tuberculosis, or regional enteritis, etc.

TECHNIQUE

AP abdomen—supine to include symphysis pubis.
AP abdomen—erect to include diaphragm.
And/or lateral abdomen—decubitus.
PA abdomen—on right and left side, decubitus.

INTRACARDIAC CALCIFICATION

Calcification of the mitral and aortic valves is not uncommon, and is a sequel to rheumatic infection, or due to atheroma.

TECHNIQUE

PA chest.
Lateral chest.
Tomography in the right anterior oblique positions.

INTUSSUSCEPTION

The invagination or passage of one part of the intestine into another, usually occurring in young infants.

TECHNIQUE

AP abdomen.
This may demonstrate absence of bowel shadows on the right side of the abdomen. Further supervised investigation involving opaque media may also be needed to confirm diagnosis.

ISCHAEMIC HEART DISEASE

This is a deficiency of the arterial blood-supply to the heart due usually to atheroma. It results in angina (q.v.) and eventually leads to local areas of myocardial fibrosis and heart failure.

TECHNIQUE

PA chest at 2 m.

JACCOUD'S ARTHRITIS

A form of peri-articular fibrosis which may occur during subsiding acute rheumatic fever. There is ulnar deviation and a flexion deformity of the metacarpophalangeal joints with subluxation of the 5th metacarpophalangeal joint and peri-articular swellings.

TECHNIQUE

PA both hands.

Norgaard's view—*see* APPENDIX.

JOHANSSON'S DISEASE

Osteochondritis of the secondary centre of ossification of the patella.

TECHNIQUE

PA both knees.

Lateral both knees.

Skyline view of both patellae.

JUNGLING'S DISEASE

See SARCOIDOSIS.

KARTAGENER'S DISEASE

An hereditary complex of symptoms consisting of bronchiectasis, sinusitis, and transposition of the viscera.

TECHNIQUE

PA chest.

Sinus views.

KIENBÖCK'S DISEASE

Osteochondritis of the semilunar (lunate) bone.

TECHNIQUE

PA both wrists.

Lateral both wrists.

KLIPPEL-FEIL SYNDROME

Congenital fusion of two or more cervical vertebrae—the spines are small and occasionally bifid—resulting in a very short neck with limited movement. Atlanto-occipital fusion is common.

TECHNIQUE

AP cervical spine.

AP upper cervical spine with jaw open or moving.

Lateral cervical spine.

KÖHLER'S DISEASE
Osteochondritis of the tarsal navicular bone and/or the head of the second metatarsal. The latter is sometimes referred to as 'Freiberg's infraction'.

TECHNIQUE
AP both feet.
Dorsiplantar oblique both feet.

KÜMMEL'S DISEASE
A post-traumatic spondylitis of the vertebrae, more common in the dorsal area.

TECHNIQUE
AP affected area.
Lateral affected area.

KYPHOSIS DORSALIS ADOLESCENTIUM
See SCHEUERMANN'S DISEASE.

KYPHOSIS DORSALIS JUVENILIS
See SCHEUERMANN'S DISEASE.

LEAD POISONING
A rare cause of poisoning, and when seen usually occurs in children who have ingested lead or its salts in some form, where it may be detected radiologically in the growing ends of the bones. This is due to the metabolism of lead being similar to that of calcium. It appears as a clear-cut band of increased density at the metaphysis of the growing bone.

TECHNIQUE
PA both wrists.
AP both ankles.

LEPROSY
A chronic infectious disease occurring in tropical and subtropical countries. The skin is most commonly involved, particularly that of the face, hands, and feet. In later stages there may be bone involvement, particularly of the metacarpals and metatarsals, where the bone increases in width with central areas of destruction.

TECHNIQUE
PA both hands.
AP both feet.
AP forearm, soft tissue—to demonstrate nerve calcification.

LETTERER-SIWE DISEASE
See HAND—SCHÜLLER—CHRISTIAN DISEASE.

LEUKAEMIA
A disease of the reticulo-endothelial system, characterized by a marked increase of the leucocytes. There are varying types but those of radiological interest are the myeloid and lymphatic types. Deposits appear in the bone in advanced cases, and are usually seen first in the long bones, with occasional osteoporosis of the skull.

TECHNIQUE
PA chest—for hilar enlargement.

AP humerus   } May demonstrate deposits in ad-
AP femur   }   vanced cases.

LIPOID GRANULOMATOSES
A term applied to a group of diseases in all of which there is a disturbance of the lipoid metabolism. This term includes such diseases as Gaucher's, Niemann—Pick, and Hand—Schüller—Christian.

TECHNIQUE
According to the type, *see under* applicable disease.

LIPOMA
A benign tumour of fat which may be multifocal, when it is known as 'Dercum's disease'. Owing to the fact that fat is slightly more translucent radiologically than the surrounding muscular tissue, it may sometimes be demonstrated as a well-defined, rounded or oval area lying between the muscular shadows.

TECHNIQUE
Lateral affected area   } To demonstrate the com-
AP affected area   }   plete range of soft-tissue
                             shadows.

LOOSE BODY IN THE KNEE
A loose body may be found in any diarthrodial joint; it has no connection with the articular surface or the lining membrane and is free to move anywhere in the joint. This is of particular clinical significance in the knee-joint, where it may cause pain and 'locking'.

TECHNIQUE
AP knee-joint.
Lateral knee-joint.
Intercondylar view.
For localization immediately prior to surgery:
AP knee-joint.
Horizontal lateral, thus maintaining the knee-joint
in the operative position.

LOOSER'S ZONES

Areas of decalcification or pseudo-fractures occurring
in osteomalacia. The characteristic occurrence
is in the lateral borders of the scapulae, pubic
rami, neck of femora, and the ribs.
See also OSTEOMALACIA.
TECHNIQUE
PA chest.
AP scapulae.
AP pelvis—to include femora.

LYMPHOSARCOMA

A malignant tumour of lymphatic tissue, with wide-
spread glandular enlargement. Radiologically the
skull may show considerable thinning at the cortex.
TECHNIQUE
AP affected area.
Lateral affected area.
PA chest.
PA skull.
Lateral skull.

MADELUNG'S DEFORMITY

This deformity is the backward projection of the
distal end of the ulna, caused by arrest in the
growth of the lower end of the radius. It is more
prevalent in females and is usually noted between
the ages of 12 and 14 years.
TECHNIQUE
Lateral of both wrists.

MADUROMYCOSIS (Mycetoma)

This is a common fungus infection occurring more
often in tropical regions. There is a direct extension
from the soft tissue myecetoma involving the bone.
The tarso-metatarsal area is the most frequently
involved, but the carpo-metacarpal area may also
be affected.

TECHNIQUE
    AP feet.
    PA hands and wrists.

MALGAIGNE'S FRACTURE

A vertical fracture of the posterior pelvic wall, on the same side, and associated with, a dislocation of the sacro-iliac joint.
TECHNIQUE
    AP pelvis—transverse stereo.

MALTA FEVER

See BRUCELLOSIS.

MARBLE BONES (Albers-Schönberg's Disease)

See OSTEOPETROSIS.

MARCH FRACTURE

Fracture of one or more metatarsal bones without obvious trauma. It is also known as a 'fatigue or stress fracture'.
TECHNIQUE
    AP foot.
    Dorsiplantar oblique.

MARFAN'S SYNDROME

See ARACHNODACTYLY.

MASTOIDITIS

An inflammation of the mastoid air-cells following infection of the middle ear.
TECHNIQUE
    Right and left lateral obliques with the pinna of the ear folded forward.
    Fronto-occipital with $30°$ caudal tilt (slit Towne's view).
    Further views as required.

MECKEL'S DIVERTICULUM

A narrow tube, blind at one end, and communicating with the lumen of the ileum at the other. It results from the failure of a duct to close during early fetal life.
TECHNIQUE
    This condition may be demonstrated by isotope imaging, but may present as an 'acute abdomen'.
    See INTESTINAL OBSTRUCTION, ACUTE.

MEDIASTINAL NEUROFIBROMA

A benign tumour of the fibrous sheath of a spinal nerve, most common in the upper dorsal area.

TECHNIQUE

PA chest.

Lateral chest.

Oblique chest.

AP dorsal spine—to show enlargement of inter-vertebral foramen.

Lateral dorsal spine.

MEDULLOBLASTOMA

A malignant tumour of the brain-stem, occurring in children. As the tumour seldom calcifies, the only radiological evidence is that of raised intracranial pressure.

TECHNIQUE

AP skull.

Lateral skull.

MEGACOLON, IDIOPATHIC

An enlargement of the colon and rectum, without the narrowed segment found in Hirschsprung's disease. Clinically it is milder and of slower onset.

TECHNIQUE

AP abdomen—erect—to show gaseous distension and splayed ends of the lower ribs.

MEIGS' SYNDROME

A combination of bilateral pleural effusion and ascites due to a fibroma of the ovary.

TECHNIQUE

PA chest.

Lateral chest.

Ultrasound abdomen or

AP abdomen with increased penetration.

MENINGIOMA

A slow-growing benign tumour of the cerebral menin-ges; radiologically it may sometimes be localized by bone sclerosis and increased blood-supply, causing more visual vascular channels.

TECHNIQUE

PA skull with 10° caudal tilt.

AP skull with 30° caudal tilt (Towne's view).

Lateral skull.

MENINGOCELE

A saccular herniation of the meninges associated with localized deficiencies of the vertebral laminae.

TECHNIQUE

AP affected area.

Lateral affected area (coned)—exposure factors selected to relate soft tissue to the vertebrae.

MENINGOMYELOCELE

A protrusion of a portion of the spinal cord membranes through a defect in the vertebral column. This can occur in any area but is more commonly seen in the lumbar spine and usually several vertebrae are involved.

TECHNIQUE

AP or PA lumbo-sacral spine (frequently more easily done PA).

Lateral if required.

MICROCEPHALY

A congenital defective development of the cerebrum with a thick skull and an early closure of the fontanelles, resulting in a small skull.

TECHNIQUE

Ultrasound.

AP skull $\left.\begin{array}{l}\\\end{array}\right\}$ for confirmation.
Lateral skull

MITRAL STENOSIS

A disease of the mitral valve of the heart, usually due to a rheumatic inflammation.

TECHNIQUE

PA chest penetrated—to show elevated left main bronchus.

Left lateral chest.

MONCKEBERG'S SCLEROSIS

A uniform calcification of the entire segment of peripheral arteries, chiefly those with a muscular coat. It does not cause completely occlusive arterial disease though it frequently co-exists with internal arterio-sclerosis.

TECHNIQUE

AP and lateral of affected area of the extremity.

MONGOLISM (Down's Syndrome)

A type of idiocy similar to that of cretinism. In the skull, the sutures often remain ununited for an unusually long time. Other bones may be found to be short for the relative age of the child, the most common site being the hands.

TECHNIQUE

PA skull.

Lateral skull.

PA both hands.

AP pelvis—to demonstrate acetabular angle.

MONTEGGIA'S DISLOCATION

The dislocation of the hip towards the anterior superior iliac spine.

TECHNIQUE

AP hip-joint.

AP hip-joint—stereo.

MONTEGGIA'S FRACTURE

A fracture of the upper shaft of the ulna associated with a dislocation of the head of the radius.

TECHNIQUE

AP forearm—to include the elbow-joint.

Lateral forearm.

MORQUIO-BRAILSFORD DISEASE *see also* MUCOPOLYSACCHARIDOSES

A type of dwarfism, often familial. It is characterized by a flattening of the vertebrae, kyphosis, progressive changes in the hip-joint and in varying degrees, deformities of all bones, except those of the face and skull. It is usually found in children, affecting particularly the epiphyses.

TECHNIQUE

Lateral cervical, dorsal and lumbar vertebrae.

AP pelvis.

MORVAN'S DISEASE

A form of syringomyelia characterized by atrophy of the digits.

TECHNIQUE

PA both hands.

MOUNIER-KUHN SYNDROME

See TRACHEOBRONCHOMEGALY.

MUCOCELE

An encysted accumulation of mucus in a gland, sinus, or organ such as the gall-bladder. Radiologically the most common sites are the ethmoid and frontal sinuses and lacrimal sac.

TECHNIQUE (for sinuses)

Occipitofrontal with $10°$ caudal tilt.

Lateral sinuses.

Right and left optic foramina views.

MUCOPOLYSACCHARIDOSES

This is a classification of certain diseases by abnormal mucopolysaccharide metabolism. It includes such conditions as Morquio-Brailsford Disease, Hunter's and Hurler's Syndrome and Gargoylism. The striking feature common to these conditions is an abnormal basic biochemistry of the skeletal system. *See* HUNTER'S SYNDROME, HURLER'S DISEASE AND MORQUIO-BRAILSFORD DISEASE.

TECHNIQUE

See synonyms for individual dysplasias.

MULTIPLE MYELOMATOSIS

A malignant growth of plasma cells, usually radiologically evident as multiple defects of the bone. The vertebral bodies are commonly affected, also the pelvis, shoulders, and skull. The distal parts of the extremities are rarely involved. Widespread, even decalcification of the vertebral column, ribs, pelvis, and proximal ends of the long bones occurs.

TECHNIQUE

Lateral spine.

AP pelvis.

AP shoulders.

Lateral skull.

PA chest.

MYECETOMA

See MADUROMYCOSIS.

MYOCARDIAL INFARCT

Death of an area of muscular tissue of the heart due to impaired circulation.

TECHNIQUE

PA chest at 2m—for heart size.

MYOSITIS

Inflammation of the muscles, of which there are several types. Only two are of radiological interest —myositis ossificans and clostridial myositis.

1. Myositis Ossificans

Bone formation in the muscle usually following trauma and/or in paraplegia, the most common sites being the distal halves of the humerus and femur.

TECHNIQUE

AP affected area.

Lateral affected area.

The exposures should be adjusted to demonstrate the muscle attachments.

2. Clostridial Myositis

Infection of the muscle by an anaerobic bacillus. This is radiologically significant by the gas infiltration outlining the muscle fibres.

TECHNIQUE

See GAS GANGRENE.

MYOSITIS PROGRESSIVA

A progressive form of myositis beginning in early life, where plaques of bone form in the fascial planes. These changes are associated with abnormalities of the thumb and great toe.

TECHNIQUE

PA both hands.

AP both feet.

NAVICULO-CUBOID BAR

A bar or bridge between the navicular and the cuboid, which can be either fibrous, cartilaginous, or osseous.

TECHNIQUE

Dorsiplantar oblique.

NEPHROBLASTOMA

See WILMS' TUMOUR.

NEPHROCALCINOSIS

A defect in the function of the renal tubules resulting in acids accumulating in the blood, and the urine containing a high proportion of calcium. Numerous small deposits of calcium are found in the medulla of the kidney.

TECHNIQUE
AP upper abdomen—for kidney outline.
(Films on inspiration and expiration and a lateral
may be required for a differential diagnosis.)

NEUROFIBROMA
A benign tumour of peripheral nerves that may be
single or multiple. Occurring at any age, they may
involve all parts of the spine, but most commonly
the thoracic region. Most of these tumours lie
between the dura and the spinal cord, but extra-
dural tumours have been found when they protrude
through and expand the intervertebral foramen,
when they are sometimes known as 'hour-glass'
tumours due to their shape.
TECHNIQUE
AP affected area.
Lateral affected area.
If they occur in the cervical or lumbar area, oblique
views are essential. If they occur in the dorsal
area, in addition to the routine AP and lateral
films an AP of the ribs should be taken to
demonstrate the head of the ribs, as there is
often a deformity and a marked deviation of
the shaft and widening of the intercostal spaces.

NIEMANN—PICK DISEASE
An acute systemic disease similar to that of Gaucher's
disease, normally occurring before the age of
2 years, causing enlargement of the liver, spleen,
and lymph nodes.
TECHNIQUE
PA chest—for rib and lung changes.
AP abdomen.

NON-ACCIDENTAL INJURY
A medico-legal problem produced by wilful trauma,
causing multiple bruising, subdural haematoma
and skeletal injuries. It occurs mainly in children
aged 0—5 years.
TECHNIQUE
AP and lateral skull.
Chest—for rib injuries.
Pelvis.

All long bones—for evidence of old fractures. In very young children one accurate projection in the AP position to include the torso and all long bones is usually acceptable.

OBSTRUCTIVE EMPHYSEMA
A partial ball valve obstruction of one of the larger bronchi. This allows air to enter the lung on inspiration but traps the air on expiration.
TECHNIQUE
PA chest on inspiration.
PA chest on expiration.

OLLIER'S DISEASE
See DYSCHONDROPLASIA.

OS ACROMIALE
An ununited acromion process, more commonly bilateral. Both shoulders should be X-rayed to differentiate between the above phenomenon and an ununited fracture.
TECHNIQUE
AP both shoulders.

OSGOOD—SCHLATTER'S DISEASE
Osteochondritis of the tibial tubercle.
TECHNIQUE
AP knee-joint.
Lateral knee-joint—both knees with slight reduction of exposure to demonstrate the tibial tubercle.

OSTEITIS DEFORMANS
See PAGET'S DISEASE.

OSTEITIS FIBROSA CYSTICA
See HYPERPARATHYROIDISM.

OSTEOCHONDRITIS
Avascular necrosis of certain ossification centres. According to their site they are known by the name of the people who discovered them.
TECHNIQUE
For lunate *see* KIENBÖCK'S DISEASE.
For second and third metatarsal heads *see* FREIBERG'S DISEASE.

For tarsal navicular *see* KÖHLER'S DISEASE.
For vertebral bodies *see* SCHEUERMANN'S DISEASE.
For tibial tubercle *see* OSGOOD–SCHLATTER'S
   DISEASE.
For patella *see* JOHANSSON'S DISEASE.
For calcaneus *see* SEVER'S DISEASE.
For head of femur *see* PERTHES' DISEASE.

OSTEOCHONDRITIS DEFORMANS JUVENILIS
See PERTHES' DISEASE.

OSTEOCHONDRITIS DEFORMANS TIBIAE
See BLOUNT'S DISEASE.

OSTEOCHONDRITIS DISSECANS
A joint infection where a necrotic process separates a
   fragment of bone lying beneath the articular carti-
   lage, which may eventually form a loose body. The
   most common site is that of the knee-joint although
   other joints may be affected.
TECHNIQUE
   AP affected area.
   Lateral affected area.
   As well as these views further projections to
      demonstrate separation of the fragment should
      be taken—these vary according to the joint.
   Knee-joint
      AP
      Lateral.
      Intercondylar view.

OSTEOCLASTOMA
See GIANT-CELL TUMOUR.

OSTEOGENESIS IMPERFECTA (Fragilitas Ossium)
A defect in bone formation and calcification characterized by bone fragility, and resulting in multiple
   fractures. Many of the fractures may have occurred
   prenatally, and throughout life fractures are con-
   tinually recurring.
TECHNIQUE
   AP affected area.
   Lateral affected area.

OSTEOID OSTEOMA
A small, circumscribed, non-inflammatory, benign
   lesion. Radiologically it appears as a translucent
   area surrounded by an exaggerated zone of sclerosis.

It is a fairly common bone lesion and may occur in any part of the skeleton, the lower extremity being the most common site.

TECHNIQUE

AP affected area.

Lateral affected area.

Tomography—this may be necessary to establish the presence of a central nidus.

OSTEOMALACIA (Adult Rickets)

A deficiency disease which radiologically shows a marked lack of calcium. It is rare in England, but may be found elsewhere, and is more common in women, when it appears to affect the pelvis first, particularly during pregnancy. Severe kypho-scoliosis may follow and deformities of the sternum and ribs, giving rise to depressions and prominences in the chest wall. *See also* LOOSER'S ZONES.

TECHNIQUE

AP pelvis.

PA chest—for ribs.

In the early stages it is helpful to obtain radiographs of a patient of similar age and size in order to demonstrate the difference in calcium density.

OSTEOMYELITIS

An acute or chronic infection causing inflammation of the bone-marrow, due to the invasion by staphylococci or streptococci. Radiological changes are not evident for at least a week after the onset of infection.

TECHNIQUE

AP affected area.

Lateral affected area.

N.B. In chronic cases an increase in penetration may be necessary.

OSTEOPETROSIS (Marble Bones)

Disturbance in bone formation which usually starts during the fetal period. All bones are affected, showing marked increase in density, but with this comes marked fragility and therefore fractures are often associated with this disease. Owing to increased density in the base of the skull, the foramen tends to become occluded.

TECHNIQUE
PA chest—for ribs.
AP pelvis.
PA skull with 10° caudal tilt.
Lateral skull.
Submento-vertical skull.
Lateral dorsal and lumbar spine.

OSTEOPOROSIS

Enlargement of the marrow and Haversian canals and a lack of bone trabeculae due to the failure of bone to produce sufficient osteoid. This may be caused by endocrine disturbance, disuse, deficiency of protein and vitamin C, or be post-traumatic (Sudeck's atrophy) or congenital (osteogenesis imperfecta). Radiologically this appears as a thinned cortex, fine or spare trabecular pattern. Fractures of the ribs and collapse of the vertebrae are quite common.
TECHNIQUE
PA chest—for ribs.
AP pelvis.
Lateral dorsal and lumbar spine.

OTOSCLEROSIS

The stapes (innermost of the ossicles) becomes fixed to the bony margin of the opening between the middle and inner ear. As a result there is ossification of the fenestra rotunda causing deafness.
TECHNIQUE
Right and left lateral obliques of the mastoid aircells—pinna of the ear folded forward.
Fronto-occipital with 35° caudal tilt (Towne's view).

OVARIAN CYSTS

A cyst or cysts in the ovaries which may be of varying types, the walls of which may calcify. When they contain teeth or hair they are known as dermoid cysts.
TECHNIQUE
AP pelvic area (with bladder empty).
For small cysts and differential diagnosis, ultrasound may be the method of choice or as an additive examination.

PAGET'S DISEASE (Osteitis Deformans)

A skeletal disease of unknown origin, characterized by slowly spreading changes in one or more bones. In the early stages the bones are porotic, but as the disease progresses the bone thickens and becomes more dense. There is complete or partial obliteration of the marrow cavity, the bone trabeculation widens and becomes more coarse. The bones soften, and bowing and flattening, particularly in weight-bearing areas, occur.

TECHNIQUE

AP skull.

Lateral skull.

AP pelvis.

AP affected area.

Lateral affected area.

PANCOAST TUMOUR (Superior Sulcus Tumour)

Carcinoma of the apex of the lung with involvement of the structures at the root of the neck, including the main nerve-trunks; it causes pain and atrophy of the muscles of the shoulder, arm, and hand. In a large number of cases erosions of the necks of the second and third ribs are visible.

TECHNIQUE

PA chest.

Lateral chest.

Apical view—plus penetration to show the ribs.

Tomography may occasionally be necessary for early diagnosis.

PANCREATITIS

Inflammation of the pancreas with possible local abscess formation.

TECHNIQUE

AP abdomen.

This may show absence of normal gas shadows and absence of gas in the mid-section of the transverse colon (Stewart's sign) or the sentinel loop, or calcification in line of pancreas.

PARALYTIC ILEUS

Atony of the intestines giving rise to obstruction and stagnation of the contents. In the erect position there is greater opacity in the lower abdomen than in the upper parts.

TECHNIQUE
AP abdomen—erect, to include diaphragm.

PARAVERTEBRAL ABSCESS
An abscess forming in the dorsal region, usually of tubercular origin.
TECHNIQUE
AP dorsal spine—on a large film, to include the whole area of the abscess shadow.

PAROSMIA
See CACOSMIA.

PATENT INTERAURICULAR DEFECT
See ATRIAL SEPTAL DEFECT.

PELLEGRINI–STIEDA LESION
Calcification of the medial collateral ligament of the knee, usually post-traumatic in origin.
TECHNIQUE
AP knee-joint.
AP knee-joint—with $10°$ external rotation of the leg, using soft-tissue technique.

PERFORATED GASTRIC or DUODENAL ULCER
An ulcer of the mucous membrane penetrating through the layers of the viscus to the peritoneum; caused by inflammation, or, in the case of gastric ulcer, sometimes by cancer.
TECHNIQUE
AP abdomen—erect, to include diaphragm.
See also INTESTINAL OBSTRUCTION, ACUTE.

PERICARDIAL ADHESIONS
Localized or generalized obliteration of the pericardial sac by an exudate or fibrosis. It may be caused by many diseases including infective pericarditis, tuberculosis, rheumatic fever, or a reaction in an area of old myocardial infarction.
TECHNIQUE
PA chest—erect.
Right lateral chest—erect.
AP chest—supine.
Right and left laterals—recumbent, on inspiration and expiration, to show any limited movement of the heart due to adhesions.

PERICARDIAL EFFUSION

An effusion accumulated in the pericardial space. Only if a sufficient amount of fluid has accumulated within this space will the radiological signs appear that can be diagnostic.

TECHNIQUE

AP chest.

Ultrasound where radiological appearances are equivocal.

PERICARDITIS

Inflammation of the pericardium, more likely to be acute than chronic. With constrictive pericarditis —a condition where there is fibrous thickening of the pericardium—there may be calcification.

TECHNIQUE

PA chest.

PA chest—penetrated, using Potter-Bucky.

Left lateral chest.

PERIRENAL ABSCESS

An abscess around the kidney, which may cause the diaphragm to show fixation on the affected side. The renal outline is obliterated and the psoas muscle may also be obliterated or displaced, and the colon altered in position.

TECHNIQUE

AP abdomen—to include the diaphragm—arrested respiration.

AP abdomen—during respiration, thus outlining the affected side due to its fixation.

PERTHES' DISEASE (Osteochondritis Deformans Juvenilis)

Osteochondritis of the head of the femur.

TECHNIQUE

AP pelvis.

AP pelvis—in frog position.

PETIT'S EVENTRATION

Unilateral congenital elevation and thinning of the diaphragm, usually on the left side.

TECHNIQUE

PA chest ⎱ It is essential for the patient
Left lateral chest ⎰ to be erect.

PLEURAL EFFUSION

Either an inflammatory exudate or transudation of fluid into the pleural sac cavity.

TECHNIQUE

PA chest

PA chest—penetrated, using Potter-Bucky

Lateral chest

} Erect or decubitus, *see* APPENDIX.

Further views according to the site may also be taken, i.e., lordotic view, tangential view.

PNEUMOCONIOSIS

Occupational disease of the lungs due to inhalation of mineral dust. Different forms are: Baritosis, Siderosis, Silicatosis, Silicosis, and Stannosis.

TECHNIQUE

PA chest.

PNEUMOPERICARDIUM

A rare condition of air within the pericardial sac, usually due to thoracic surgical procedure or an artificial pneumothorax.

TECHNIQUE

PA chest with full inspiration and expiration (for a differential diagnosis between pneumopericardium and a mediastinal hernia).

PNEUMOPERITONEUM

Free gas in the peritoneal cavity, which may result from a laparotomy, perforation of the alimentary canal, gas-forming abscesses, or may be artificially induced.

TECHNIQUE

AP abdomen—erect, to include diaphragm, or

PA abdomen—decubitus, lying on the left side (the left side is best to demonstrate free gas under the right dome of the diaphragm, as it contains no gut). *See* APPENDIX.

PNEUMOTHORAX

A condition where air or other gas is present in the pleural cavity, resulting in collapse of the lung. This may be produced artificially for medical reasons or may have occurred spontaneously.

TECHNIQUE
>AP or PA chest—erect (where it is difficult to diagnose, films on inspiration and expiration and stereos may be taken).
>AP decubitus with affected side up in the new-born or injured child.

POLYDACTYLY
The presence of extra digits or parts of digits.
TECHNIQUE
>PA both hands.

POPLITEAL BURSITIS (Baker's Cyst)
Inflammation and fluid forming as a result of an infective process. It occurs mainly in the elderly and may be accompanied by a calcified popliteal artery.
TECHNIQUE
>Lateral knee—with horizontal beam to show cyst within the popliteal space.

POST-CRICOID CARCINOMA
A tumour of the pharynx which has an early lymphatic spread. There is a swelling opposite the lower cervical vertebrae with forward displacement of the trachea.
TECHNIQUE
>Lateral neck—soft tissue with Valsalva's manœuvre. (*See* APPENDIX.)
>Tomography.

POTT'S DISEASE
Tuberculosis of the spine.
TECHNIQUE
>AP affected area.
>Lateral affected area.
>It is important, when examining these cases, to include in the technique an AP on a large film so that the presence of either a paravertebral or psoas abscess, dependent on the area, may be detected.

PROTRUSIO ACETABULAE
A softening of the bones of the acetabulum, which becomes deepened due to the pressure from the head of the femur.
TECHNIQUE
>AP pelvis.

PSEUDO-GOUT
See CHONDROCALCINOSIS.

PSOAS ABSCESS
An abscess forming in the psoas muscle, usually of
tuberculous origin.
TECHNIQUE
AP abdomen—to include thoracic vertebra 11 to
the lesser trochanters of the femora—its origin
and insertion.

PSORIATIC ARTHRITIS
When arthritis is seen combined with psoriasis it
usually affects the interphalangeal joints as well as
the metacarpophalangeal joints and the wrists, as
in rheumatoid arthritis. There is a narrowing of the
affected joint space and marginal splaying at the
base of the phalanges.
TECHNIQUE
PA hands.
Laterals of both feet—for involvement of the
plantar aspect of the calcaneum.

PULMONARY EMBOLISM
A pulmonary embolism without infarction is difficult
to recognize on a plain radiograph. Occasionally the
hilar shadow on the affected side may be enlarged
and there may also be local areas of hyperlucency
(Westermark's sign).
TECHNIQUE
PA chest.
Lateral chest (with infarction).

PULMONARY STENOSIS
A narrowing of the valve of the pulmonary artery,
where it arises from the right ventricle (pulmonary
conus).
TECHNIQUE
PA chest.
Left and right anterior oblique.

PYOPNEUMOTHORAX
A mixture of pus and air present in the pleural cavity.
If this is localized at the base of the lung it is
difficult to differentiate from a subphrenic abscess.

TECHNIQUE
AP or PA chest—with patient lying on the left side.
Lateral chest—supine.

RAISED INTRACRANIAL PRESSURE
When the intracranial pressure is raised for any length of time, there is engorgement of the emissary veins enlarging the channels where they perforate the skull near the occipital protuberance. The meningeal vessels may also enlarge, increasing the size of the foramen spinosum. There is also erosion of the posterior clinoid processes, an increase in size of the pituitary fossa and loss of the floor. In children there is diastasis of the sutures.
TECHNIQUE
AP skull with $35°$ caudal tilt (Towne's view).
PA skull with $10°$ caudal tilt.
Submento-vertical view.
Lateral skull.
Coned pituitary fossa.

RATHKE'S POUCH TUMOUR
See CRANIOPHARYNGIOMA.

RAYNAUD'S DISEASE
Spasm of peripheral arteries due to cold; it may eventually proceed to gangrene of the finger-tips.
TECHNIQUE
PA both hands—to include tufts of the terminal phalanges.

REITER'S DISEASE
An infective condition with the triad of arthritis, conjunctivitis, and urethritis. The causative agent is not known.
TECHNIQUE
AP pelvis—to show sclerosis of lower segment of sacro-iliac joints.
Lateral calcaneus—to show roughening of plantar aspect of calcaneal spur.

RENAL CALCULUS
Solid bodies formed by salts precipitated from the urine. These may form in the kidney, ureter, or bladder.

TECHNIQUE
AP abdomen.
Lateral abdomen.
For differential diagnosis films on inspiration and expiration may be taken, the patient's bowels having been adequately prepared.

RENAL CARBUNCLE
An inflammatory lesion, which deteriorates into small, multiple abscess cavities, producing soft-tissue swelling.
TECHNIQUE
AP abdomen—for renal outline.

RENAL OSTEOSCLEROSIS (Osteodystrophy)
A generalized increase in the bone density throughout the axial skeleton. This is secondary to the failure of the kidney to excrete calcium and phosphorus. Areas of increased density are seen, particularly in the submetaphysial region of the long bones.
TECHNIQUE
AP long bones, upper and lower limbs.
AP spine—to show 'rugger jersey effect'.

RETROPHARYNGEAL ABSCESS
An abscess arising behind the pharynx, caused by various diseases, such as Pott's disease or lymphadenitis.
TECHNIQUE
Lateral soft tissue of the neck to define fluid levels (Valsalva's manœuvre—*see* APPENDIX.)

RETROSTERNAL GOITRE
Either a downward growth of the thyroid gland from a cervical goitre, until it extends under the sternum, or a separate development within the thorax. May become radiologically apparent by indentation or displacement of the air-filled trachea.
TECHNIQUE
PA chest.
PA thoracic inlet—with
Valsalva's manœuvre
Lateral thoracic inlet—flying
angel technique

See APPENDIX.

RHEUMATIC HEART DISEASE

A disease of the heart following rheumatic fever. The pericardium, myocardium, and endocardium are damaged, and areas of fibrosis occur, also stenosis of the mitral and aortic valves.

TECHNIQUE

PA chest at 2 m—for heart size.

RHEUMATOID ARTHRITIS

A chronic arthritis of unknown aetiology. It usually starts gradually, but may be of sudden onset accompanied by general symptoms, such as fever, leucocytosis, anaemia, etc. Most frequently involved are the small joints of the hands and feet followed by the larger joints.

(*See also* STILL'S DISEASE.)

TECHNIQUE

AP feet.

PA hands.

AP hands in 'ball-catching' position or tangential position—to demonstrate antero-lateral aspect of metacarpal heads.

Brewerton's view ⎫
Norgaard's view ⎬ *See* APPENDIX.

RICKETS

A deficiency of the growing osteoid tissue with impaired calcification and bone formation. This is due primarily to a lack of vitamin D. The principal changes occur in the metaphyses, giving the bone ends a splayed appearance which in more advanced cases becomes a saucer deformity.

TECHNIQUE

PA both wrists.

AP both ankles.

AP both knees.

PA chest—for splaying of the anterior ends of the ribs.

ROWAN WILLIAMS'S SIGN

The great vessels of the fetus containing gas, denoting fetal death in utero.

TECHNIQUE

See FETAL DEATH IN UTERO.

RUPTURED DIAPHRAGM

Usually due to trauma. If a pneumothorax and a pneumoperitoneum exist this is proof that the diaphragm is torn, 95% of these cases occur on the left side.

TECHNIQUE

PA chest—penetrated.

PA chest ⎫
AP abdomen ⎭ Erect or decubitus.

(For minimal rupture, AP chest sitting and Trendelenburg to produce herniation.)

RUPTURED OESOPHAGUS

Usually a longitudinal tear in the lower third of the thoracic portion, the causes of which may be traumatic, secondary to ulceration, or neoplasm.

TECHNIQUE

PA chest—to include neck to show emphysema.

Lateral chest.

If several hours have elapsed since suspected rupture, a thin air line may become evident along the outer cardiac border, and a hydropneumothorax may be present; this requires: PA chest—penetrated, using Potter-Bucky.

RUPTURED SPLEEN

Usually of traumatic origin. It may cause dilatation of the stomach and a deep serration of the greater curvature. The splenic flexure of the colon may be depressed together with an immobility of the left dome of the diaphragm.

TECHNIQUE

AP abdomen—to include the diaphragm.

AP abdomen—to include diaphragm—during respiration.

SABRE TIBIA

Periosteal reaction due to congenital syphilis causing widening of the tibia on the convexity of the diaphysis.

TECHNIQUE

Laterals both tibiae.

SALIVARY CALCULI

A formation of stones in the glands and their ducts which may contain calcium salts and will, therefore, be radio-opaque.

TECHNIQUE
Parotid Gland and Stenson's Duct
PA
True lateral.
Submandibular Gland and Wharton's Duct
Lateral oblique.
True lateral, with tongue depressed.
Sublingual Gland
Lateral oblique (patient rotated towards symphysis menti).
Intra-oral.

SARCOIDOSIS (Besnier-Boeck Disease or Jungling's Disease)

An inflammatory disease of unknown origin which may attack any part of the body, either in single or multiple areas, the most common site being the hands.
TECHNIQUE
PA chest—for lungs and hilar region.
PA hands—for cysts in the phalanges.

SARCOMA OF THE SKULL

Rapidly growing malignant tumour. New spicules of bone are laid down at right-angles to the bone surface and not always visualized with standard penetration.
TECHNIQUE
Routine skull views.
Tangential views with soft radiation.

SCABBARD TRACHEA

Bilateral compression of the trachea due to an enlarged thyroid gland.
TECHNIQUE
PA thoracic inlet—with Valsalva's manœuvre
Lateral thoracic inlet—flying angel technique
} *See* APPENDIX.

SCHEUERMANN'S DISEASE

Osteochondritis of the vertebral epiphyseal plates mainly occurring in the dorsal spine, particularly the lower vertebrae, causing dorsal kyphosis. The radiographic appearance is that of wedging of the vertebral bodies.

TECHNIQUE
Lateral dorsal spine——to demonstrate articular surfaces. (Exposure factors should be recorded for repeat examinations.)

SCHISTOSOMIASIS (Bilharziasis)
This disease is an infestation by a worm which completes the other half of its life cycle in a snail and which is acquired by man through the skin from water infected with the eggs. It is a tropical disease and endemic in Asia and Africa. It causes a dermatitis and also infiltration of viscera, especially the urinary bladder, sometimes resulting in calcification of that organ.

TECHNIQUE
AP bladder with 15° caudal tilt.

SCHLATTER'S DISEASE
See OSGOOD–SCHLATTER'S DISEASE

SCHMORL'S NODES
Herniation of the nucleus pulposus into the vertebral body, occurring mainly in the dorsal and lumbar spine. The radiographic appearance shows 'punched-out' areas in the vertebral body.

TECHNIQUE
Lateral area concerned.

SCHÜLLER'S DISEASE
See HAND–SCHÜLLER–CHRISTIAN DISEASE.

SCLERODERMA
A systemic condition, mild in onset, characterized by firm, non-pitting oedema, pigmentation, weight-loss, and muscle atrophy. As a result of the muscle atrophy, there may be fibrosis of the lungs and the oesophagus may become shortened and thickened particularly at the distal end. Effusions may occur in the lungs and joint spaces. A common manifestation of this condition is the absorption of the tip of one or more terminal phalanges. There may also be associated areas of calcification in the pulp of the finger-tips.

TECHNIQUE
PA chest—for heart size and effusions.
Lateral chest.
PA hands—to include terminal tufts.
Individual laterals of fingers.

SCOLIOSIS

Lateral curvature of the spine, the degree of which may vary during growth, needing continuous surveillance.

TECHNIQUE

AP whole spine—erect—to include iliac crests on one film.

Follow-up films should be identical in position so that they may be superimposed and the degree of curvature measured.

Some centres are using PA technique combined with the use of an air gap to decrease the dose to breast tissue, in particular in the young age groups.

SCURVY

Vitamin-C deficiency. The areas most commonly affected are the lower ends of the humerus, femur, tibia, and radius. The metaphysis shows loss of density and the epiphysis presents a 'ground-glass' appearance (Wimberger's sign).

TECHNIQUE

AP and lateral of one of each of the following joints: elbow, knee, ankle, wrist.

PA chest—to demonstrate anterior ends of the ribs.

SESAMOIDITIS

Inflammation of the sesamoid bones, the first meta-tarsophalangeal joint being the most common site.

TECHNIQUE

Lateral foot.

Axial view—*See* APPENDIX.

SEVER'S DISEASE

Osteochondritis of the calcaneal epiphysis.

TECHNIQUE

Lateral both calcanei.

SICKLE CELL DISEASE

A chronic haemolytic anaemia of congenital and hereditary origin. The disease occurs almost exclusively in the black races. There are characteristic radiological changes of marrow hyperplasia, endosteo apposition of bone, bone infarction and possibly super-added infection. Common areas of

infarction are the femoral heads and the vertebral bodies.
TECHNIQUE
AP of affected area.
Lateral views as required.

SPALDING'S SIGN
The overlap and disalignment of the cranial bones due to the shrinkage of the cerebrum. This is a sign of fetal death in utero.
TECHNIQUE
See FETAL DEATH IN UTERO.

SPINA BIFIDA OCCULTA
The defective development of the spinal canal occurring in any part of the spinal column, but most commonly in the lumbosacral region.
TECHNIQUE
AP area affected.

SPINA VENTOSA
See DACTYLITIS.

SPLENIC CALCIFICATION
This condition may result from abscess formation, infarct, or tuberculosis, and is common in old age.
TECHNIQUE
AP left upper abdomen.
Lateral left upper abdomen.

SPLENOMEGALY
An enlargement of the spleen, which is a common accompaniment of many diseases of the lymphatic and reticulo-endothelial systems, also of congestive heart failure, portal hypertension, and certain anaemias and leukaemias.
TECHNIQUE
AP abdomen—erect, to include diaphragm.
PA chest.

SPONDYLITIS ANKYLOPOIETICA
See also ANKYLOSING SPONDYLITIS, BAMBOO SPINE.
A chronic inflammatory condition involving the spinal ligaments, the most common site of onset being the sacro-iliac joints and the lower lumbar spine.
TECHNIQUE
See under ANKYLOSING SPONDYLITIS.

SPONDYLOLISTHESIS

The forward displacement of a vertebra upon the one below, the commonest site being between the sacrum and 5th lumbar vertebra.

TECHNIQUE

AP and lateral area concerned.

Lumbosacral region

AP with knees flexed.

Lateral.

Oblique views with 10° cephalic tilt (to project 5th lumbar vertebra above iliac crest).

SPONTANEOUS PNEUMOTHORAX

See PNEUMOTHORAX.

SPRENGEL'S DEFORMITY

A congenital deformity of the scapula, which may be uni- or bilateral, producing an abnormally high scapula which may be united with the cervical vertebrae.

TECHNIQUE

AP both shoulders on one film.

SPRUE

See STEATORRHOEA, IDIOPATHIC.

STEATORRHOEA, IDIOPATHIC

Profuse fatty stools due to inability of the intestines to absorb fat. It is also characterized by disturbance of calcium metabolism and severe anaemia.

TECHNIQUE

AP abdomen

AP pelvis—to include femoral neck   } to demonstrate osteo-malacia.

Ribs

STILL'S DISEASE

Onset of chronic polyarthritis before the age of 16, sometimes demonstrated by the tendency to bony fusion, particularly of carpus and tarsus, and growth anomalies of fingers and toes.

TECHNIQUE

AP and lateral feet.

PA hands.

AP affected area.

SUBACROMIAL CALCIFICATION

Calcification of either tendinous cuff or subacromial bursa.

TECHNIQUE

AP shoulder.

AP shoulder with $25-30°$ caudal tilt.

SUBAORTIC STENOSIS

Narrowing of the aorta at its origin. There may be associated calcification of the aortic ring and valves with an enlargement of the ascending aorta and high aortic knuckle.

TECHNIQUE

PA chest.

Right and left anterior obliques.

SUBLUXATION OF THE ACROMIOCLAVICULAR JOINT

A partial dislocation of the acromioclavicular joint. In these cases the coracoid and trapezoid ligaments remain intact. The condition becomes more apparent with weight-bearing.

TECHNIQUE

AP both acromioclavicular joints, with patient in lordotic position. (Both joints on 43×18 cm or two 16×22 cm with one exposure. Repeat with equal weight-bearing.)

AP shoulder-joint.

SUBLUXATION OF THE KNEE-JOINT

An incomplete dislocation of the knee-joint.

TECHNIQUE

AP knee.

Lateral knee.

Lateral knee, weight-bearing—*see* APPENDIX.

SUBPHRENIC ABSCESS

An abscess below the diaphragm which may be associated with fluid levels and the presence of gas.

TECHNIQUE

AP abdomen—erect (to include diaphragm).

PA abdomen—in right decubitus position, if patient cannot be placed erect (*see* APPENDIX.)

Ultrasound.

SUDECK'S ATROPHY

An acute bone atrophy secondary to trauma, often minor, manifested on a radiograph by marked 'thinning' and mottling of the bone.

TECHNIQUE

Affected area and corresponding unaffected area for comparison.

SUPERIOR SULCUS TUMOUR

See PANCOAST TUMOUR.

SUPRARENAL CALCIFICATION

This may be caused by tuberculous infection but can be neonatal or haemorrhagic in origin.

TECHNIQUE

AP upper abdomen
Right and left obliques
} (Varied phases of respiration should be used for differential diagnosis.)

SUPRASPINATUS CALCIFICATION

See CALCAREOUS TENDINITIS.

SYNDACTYLY

A congenital abnormality of web fingers and toes which may be combined with bony fusion.

TECHNIQUE

AP feet.
PA hands.

SYPHILITIC AORTITIS

A syphilitic infection of the walls of the thoracic aorta, often associated with similar infection of the aortic valves, causing irregular dilatations in the walls of the vessel.

TECHNIQUE

PA chest.
Left anterior oblique chest.

SYRINGOMYELIA

A cavitation occurring in the centre of the spinal cord. Usually cervical and upper dorsal area. The disease is of unknown origin and usually occurs in adult life. Charcot's joints and claw feet occur.

TECHNIQUE
AP cervical spine—to show widening of the pedicles.
Joints of upper limb.
AP feet.
Lateral feet.

TALIPES

Any one of a variety of deformities of the feet, especially those of congenital origin. When using the following techniques it may be necessary to include the other foot for comparison.

1. **Talipes Calcaneocavus**
   Dorsal rotation of the calcaneus, and plantar tilting of the forefoot.
   TECHNIQUE
   Lateral foot and ankle.
   Lateral foot and ankle, weight-bearing.

2. **Talipes Calcaneovalgus**
   Calcaneal deformity with valgus deviation.
   TECHNIQUE
   AP foot with 30° cephalic tilt.

3. **Talipes Cavus (Claw Foot)**
   Increased curvature of the forefoot.
   TECHNIQUE
   Lateral foot and ankle.
   Lateral foot and ankle, weight-bearing.

4. **Talipes Equinovarus (Club Foot)**
   Deformity of extreme inversion of the foot with weight falling on the outer border and with an associated rotation and adduction.
   TECHNIQUE
   AP foot with 30° cephalic tilt.
   Lateral foot and ankle.
   Lateral foot and ankle, weight-bearing.

5. **Talipes Equinus**
   Heel is elevated with weight thrown on to the forefoot.
   TECHNIQUE
   AP foot with 30° cephalic tilt.
   Lateral foot and ankle.
   Lateral foot and ankle, weight-bearing.

6. **Talipes Planus (Flat Foot)**
   The condition of flat foot.

TECHNIQUE
Lateral foot and ankle.
Lateral foot and ankle, weight-bearing.

7. **Talipes Valgus**
The outer border of the foot is everted, and there is inward rotation of the tarsus and flattening of the plantar arch.
TECHNIQUE
AP foot with $30°$ cephalic tilt.

8. **Talipes Varus**
The foot is inverted with weight falling on the outer border.
TECHNIQUE
AP foot with $30°$ cephalic tilt.
Lateral foot and ankle.
Lateral foot and ankle, weight bearing.

TALOCALCANEAL BAR
A bar or bridge between the talus and calcaneus, being either fibrous, cartilaginous, or osseous in nature.
TECHNIQUE
Dorsiplantar oblique foot.
Lateral foot.
Axial view of the calcaneus with increased penetration.

THALASSAEMIA MAJOR (Cooley's Anaemia)
A congenital haemolytic anaemia which causes erythropoietic hyperplasia. There is a widening of the diploë of the skull and in later stages the outer table throws out bony spicules. The vertebrae are osteoporotic and coarsely trabeculated. The ribs develop an expansion of the bone structures due to marrow hypertrophy and the femora become flask-shaped. Changes may be seen in all bones in infants and children.
TECHNIQUE (In Adults)
Lateral skull.
AP and lateral spine.
AP pelvis.

THYMUS, ENLARGEMENT OF
An enlargement of lymphoid and epithelial structure in the thymus which is normally prominent in childhood, and undergoes atrophy in adult life.

TECHNIQUE
> PA chest—on full inspiration, to avoid confusion with dilated greater vessels.
>
> Lateral chest—to include 7th cervical vertebra—to cover full extension of gland. (Flying angel technique—*see* APPENDIX.)
>
> Lateral tomograms of the anterior mediastinum (in an adult).

TIETZE'S DISEASE (Costal chondritis)

An idiopathic inflammatory swelling most frequently involving the costochondral junction at the level of the 2nd anterior rib. A soft tissue mass is usually present in the early stages. The affected cartilage may eventually calcify and periosteal reaction can develop causing an increase in the size and density of the affected rib.

TECHNIQUE
> PA chest for differential diagnosis.
>
> Tangential view of soft tissue mass when present.

TOXOPLASMOSIS

An infectious disease caused by a parasite carried by animals. It occurs mainly in children and may affect the brain, causing convulsions. Specks of calcification may occur. This disease is transmitted in utero.

TECHNIQUE
> PA skull.
>
> Lateral skull.

TRACHEOBRONCHOMEGALY (Mounier-Kuhn's syndrome)

A possible familial condition characterized by dilatation of the trachea and major bronchi due to congenital weakness of the elastic and muscular fibres in the tracheobronchial tree.

TECHNIQUE
> PA chest—penetrated to show increased diameter of the trachea.
>
> Lateral chest.

TRIAL OF LABOUR

Radiographs are sometimes required to help assess the moulding of the fetal head, and whether it has become engaged.

TECHNIQUE
Lateral pelvis.
Lateral pelvis—decubitus, with feet tilted down 35° to assess if the head is engaged.

TRUNCUS ARTERIOSUS

A congenital fault in the heart whereby a single vessel arises from both ventricles above a septal defect.
TECHNIQUE
PA chest.
Left anterior oblique.

TURNER'S SYNDROME

A chromosomal disorder more common in girls. The syndrome is comprised of agenesis of the gonads, short stature, webbing of the neck and cubitus valgus. There may also be other congenital abnormalities such as co-arctation of the aorta.
TECHNIQUE
AP clavicles.
AP ribs.
PA hands and wrists (for short 4th metacarpal).
AP and lateral knees—for overgrowth and notching of the femoral condyle and depression of the tibial condyles.

ULNAR NERVE PALSY

A lesion of the ulnar nerve often associated with bone injury owing to its superficial course in the region of the elbow and wrist, resulting in a traumatic ulnar neuritis.
TECHNIQUE
According to area of pain
  Elbow
    PA
    Lateral.
    Ulnar groove view (*see* APPENDIX).
  Wrist
    PA
    Lateral.
    Carpal tunnel view (*see* APPENDIX).

UNDULANT FEVER
See BRUCELLOSIS.

VERTICAL TALUS
Congenital malposition of the talus.
TECHNIQUE
AP feet, weight-bearing.
Lateral feet, weight-bearing.
Lateral feet in the neutral position (non-weight-bearing).

VIBRATION SYNDROME
See DRILLER'S DISEASE.

VOLKMANN'S CONGENITAL ANKLE DEFORMITY
A condition where, although the foot is normal, it is in the valgus position. The fibula is only rudimentary and the ankle lies obliquely.
TECHNIQUE
AP both ankles.

WILMS' TUMOUR (Nephroblastoma)
A rare tumour of the kidney usually occurring in the first 7 years of life. There are widespread metastases—the lung is the most common site.
TECHNIQUE
AP abdomen ⎫
Lateral abdomen ⎬ to show the kidney outline.
PA chest.
Ultrasound examination of the kidney.

WIMBERGER'S SIGN
An appearance occurring in scurvy. Radiologically it is an area of irregular density in the epiphysis forming a ring about the nucleus which is more translucent than normal. It is best seen in the bones of the tarsus, particularly those of the astragalus and calcaneus. It is not a sign of active disease as it remains apparent several years after the arrest of the disease.
TECHNIQUE
Lateral foot and ankle.

YAWS
An infectious, non-venereal disease occurring in tropical climates. Bone lesions only occur in later stages of the disease, and radiologically have similar appearances to that of tertiary syphilis. It is unusual for many bones to be affected and is usually found in the long bones, presenting an appearance of areas of rarefaction. In the tertiary

stage there may be cortical destruction, with necrosis of the cancellous bone and adjacent soft tissue giving rise to ulcers.

TECHNIQUE

AP affected area.

Lateral affected area.

APPENDIX

BICIPITAL GROOVE

Patient stands with palm of hand of affected side against the side of the thigh, the body inclined forward. Tilt tube forward in same direction, central ray through long axis of bicipital groove.

BOHLER'S ANGLE

The angle formed by the upper margin of the tuberosity of the calcaneus and the subtalar joint— usually $140°$—but in severe injuries the angle may become a straight line.

TECHNIQUE

True lateral of the tarsus.

BONE AGE

Assessment of skeletal development during the years of growth is usually performed by comparing a film of the left hand and wrist with standards for each sex, as illustrated by Greulich and Pyle (1959). Accelerated or retarded maturation may be a valuable diagnostic indication, especially in metabolic bone disease. Correlation of the bone age with chronological age and height may enable a reasonably accurate forecast of mature height to be made.

TECHNIQUE

PA left hand and wrist.

BREWERTON'S VIEW

A tangential view to demonstrate the metacarpal heads and bases of the proximal phalanges, particularly useful in demonstrating early rheumatoid arthritis.

TECHNIQUE

The dorsal aspect of the digits are placed in contact with the film, thumb everted and hand flexed $60°$ at the metacarpophalangeal joints. The X-ray tube is tilted $15°$ transversely towards the radial side of the hand and centred over the ulnar side of the 3rd metacarpal.

CARPAL TUNNEL VIEW

Wrist dorsiflexed to $35°$ or more, over a support.
Tube horizontal, directed through the carpal tunnel.
Film at right-angles to central beam.
Both wrists for comparison.

DECUBITUS TECHNIQUE

AP or lateral films taken with patient in horizontal position, central ray directed horizontally to film.

FLYING ANGEL TECHNIQUE

Patient erect, arms and shoulders drawn down and right back, chin fully extended.

GRICE OPERATION

Triple arthrodesis of the tarsal bones—calcaneum/talus/navicular.

TECHNIQUE

True lateral of tarsus.

AP with cephalic tilt.

45° oblique.

JUDET'S VIEW

To demonstrate pelvic osteoma or fracture of the ischial/ischium area.

TECHNIQUE

45° right and left obliques of the side affected.

LIMB MEASUREMENT

Method 1—Scanning

TECHNIQUE

Reduce diaphragm aperture to 3 mm wide at right-angles to longitudinal axis of the limb.

During the exposure the tube is moved over the entire limb for a period of 8—10 s—slowing the speed over the thicker areas to produce an even film density.

Special 35·6 × 91·4 cm cassettes and film can be obtained, or films placed end to end.

Method 2—With Marker

TECHNIQUE

Patient supine—pelvis must be as symmetrical as possible. Place ruler marker (special ruler or long, narrow metal strip marked out at 1-cm intervals) between the legs to extend from the hips to the ankle-joints.

With patient maintained in this position without movement

Three exposures on one 35 × 43 cm film divided horizontally into three parts by lead strips.

First exposure of hip-joints, centre at level of joints.

Second exposure of knee-joints, moving film and tube, centre at level of joints.

Third exposure of ankle-joints, moving film and tube, centre at level of joints.

MACQUET VIEW
AP long leg film from hip to ankle inclusive.

MAMMOGRAPHY
The above examination can be used to assist in the diagnosis and localization of breast tumours, and in the follow-up of cases where radiotherapy and endocrine surgery have taken place. Considerable attention must be given to every radiographic factor to obtain films of the highest quality.

TECHNIQUE

Craniocaudal view.

Mediolateral view.

Axial view, patient AP and rotated 30° to lateral. Humerus lying at right-angles to the body.

NORGAARD'S VIEW
This view is also known as the 'ball catching technique', and as with Brewerton's View is useful in demonstrating early rheumatoid arthritis. It also demonstrates both the triquetrum and pisiform which are subject to early erosion in rheumatoid arthritis.

TECHNIQUE

The palms of both hands are placed face upwards in a cupping position suitable for catching a ball, with the dorsal aspect of the hand in contact with the film. Centre midway between both hands on a level with the midshaft of the 5th metacarpals.

SESAMOID BONES
Axial View of First Metatarsophalangeal Joint
Patient sitting with leg extended, film held firmly against and at right-angles to the instep. Flexion of the joint is assisted by a bandage held taut around the digit of the great toe.

Centre over the sesamoid bones at right-angles to film.

SKELETAL SURVEY
For generalized disease
TECHNIQUE
AP long bones unilaterally.
Lateral skull.
AP pelvis.
AP and lateral spine.

STENVER'S PROJECTION
Patient in PA position, head rotated 45° towards affected side.
Orbitomeatal line perpendicular to the film.
Central ray directed to external occipital protuberance with tube angled 12° caudally.

STRYKER'S PROJECTION
Patient supine, affected arm raised, palm of hand placed on the back of the head.
Tube tilt of 10° cephalad centred through shoulder-joint.

SUBLUXATION OF KNEE-JOINT
Lateral View—Weight-bearing
Patient standing with sound limb forward in relaxed position.
Affected limb fully extended taking full weight of body.
Film supported vertically against lateral aspect of knee.
Centre with tube horizontal to medial tuberosity of tibia.

ULNAR GROOVE PROJECTION
Patient sitting or PA prone, with elbow PA and flexed to 35° over frame or pad.
Tube horizontal, directed through groove, which is easily palpated.
Film resting on dorsal aspect of the humerus at right-angles to central beam.
Both sides for comparison.

VALSALVA'S MANŒUVRE
Deep inspiration, close mouth and nose, and forcibly expire against closure.

VON ROSEN'S PROJECTION

This technique needs absolute accuracy and should be supervised by a qualified medical practitioner. The patient should be held in the true AP position with the femora abducted 45° and firmly internally rotated 45°. In the resultant radiograph a line through both the shafts of the femora should meet at the L5/S1 junction.

BIBLIOGRAPHY

Aegerter E. and Kirkpatrick J. A. (1963) *Physiology, Pathology, and Radiology of Orthopedic Diseases*, Philadelphia: Saunders.

Anderson W. A. D. (1952) *Synopsis of Pathology*, London: Kimpton.

Boyd W. (1961) *Textbook of Pathology*, 7th ed. London: Kimpton.

Brews A. (1963) *Manual of Obstetrics*, 12th ed. London: Churchill.

Caffey J. (1967) *Paediatric X-ray Diagnosis*, 5th ed. Chicago: Year Book Publishers.

Caffey J. (1978) *Paediatric X-ray Diagnosis* I and II, 7th ed., Year Book Publishers.

Clarke K. C. (1956) *Positioning in Radiography*, London: Heinemann.

Davies P. M. (1960) *Medical Terminology for Radiographers*, London: Heinemann.

Davies W. G. (1965) Radiography of Congenital and Acquired Deformities of the Foot. In: *X-ray Focus*, Vol. 6, No. 1. Ilford.

Drummond A. and Osborne M. A. (1973) Early Detection of Rheumatoid Arthritis. In: *X-ray Focus*, Vol. 12, No. 3. Ilford.

Egan R. L. (1966) Technical Aspects of Mammography. In: *Medical Radiography and Photography*, Vol. 42, No. 1. Rochester, N.Y.

Gordon I. R. S. and Ross S. G. M. (1977) *Diagnostic Radiology in Paediatrics*, London: Butterworths.

Greulich W. W. and Pyle S. I. (1959) *Radiographic Atlas of Skeletal Development of the Hand and Wrist*, London: Oxford University Press.

Hartley J. B. and Fisher A. S. (1966) *A Plan for Radiography in Obstetrics*, Manchester: Jesse Broad.

Lewis T. L. T. (1964) *Progress in Clinical Obstetrics and Gynaecology*, 2nd ed. London: Churchill.

Lodge T. (1964) *Recent Advances in Radiology*, 4th ed. London: Churchill.

Shanks S. C. and Kerley P. (1962) *A Textbook of X-ray Diagnosis*, London: Lewis.

Shutliffe E. E. (1962) *Children's Radiographic Technique,* 2nd ed. London: Kimpton.

Simons S. (1965) *Principles of Bone X-ray Diagnosis,* 2nd ed. London: Butterworths.

Simpson C. K. (1973) *Child Abuse— The Battered Baby.* London: Butterworths.

Stripp W. J. (1963) Radiography of the Shoulder. In: *X-ray Focus,* Vol. 4, No. 2. Ilford.

Stripp W. J. (1963) Radiography of the Shoulder. In: *X-ray Focus,* Vol. 4, No. 3. Ilford.

Stripp W. J. (1964) Radiography of the Shoulder. In: *X-ray Focus,* Vol. 5, No. 1. Ilford.

Stripp W. J. (1964) Radiography of the Shoulder. In: *X-ray Focus,* Vol. 5, No. 2. Ilford.

Stripp W. J. (1966) Radiography of the Knee Joint. In: *X-ray Focus,* Vol. 7, No. 3. Ilford.

Sutton D. (1980) *Textbook of Radiology and Imaging* Vol. I and II, 3rd ed. London: Churchill Livingstone.